M

PREGNANCY
Beth Wilson Saavedra

WORKMAN PUBLISHING, NEW YORK

Cover illustration by Lori Sue Johnson

Library of Congress Cataloging-in-Publication Data

Saavedra, Beth Wilson.
Meditations during pregnancy / by Beth Wilson Saavedra.
    p. cm.
ISBN 0-7611-1995-7 (pbk. : alk. paper)
    1. Mothers—Prayer-books and devotions—English.
    2. Pregnancy—Religious aspects. I. Title.
BL625.68 .S32 2001
618.2'4—dc21   2001033323

Workman Publishing
708 Broadway
New York, NY 10003

Printed in the United States

First printing August 2001

10 9 8 7 6 5 4 3 2

To my son Alexander, I give the deepest bow of thanks. Your very presence in my life has made me reach more deeply into my essence, strength, patience, vision, and laughter. You have helped me to grow, and grow up. I love you, my dear, sweet child. May you always know your worth. The angels and I adore you.

To all the mothers of the world and all the soon-to-be mothers, value the contributions you make; they are a sacred gift to the next generation.

J am incredibly lucky to have so many wonderful people in my life . . .

To my mother, Anne, I thank you for showing me the world and the many possibilities that exist "outside the box."

To my father, Paul, and my mother, Linda, thank you so much for coming through for Alexander and me when we needed you most. You are great grandparents!

To my grandparents: I would not be who I am had I not received so much from each of you. I miss you and wish my child could have known you.

I extend a big thank-you to my uncle Brian and his wonderful wife, Beth. I could not ask for two more honest, loving, and funny people in my family. Glad I have relatives like you!

To my aunt Sylvia for all her kind and encouraging words. Thank you.

To Jon, Matt, and Sara, thank you for being you. I have learned so much from each of you. Big hugs and much love. And to the George family—Joann, Mario, Vera, Dave, Diane, John, Cindy, and Rob, thank you for opening your hearts.

I have the most incredible, courageous, generous, loving, and sassy friends. I love you all: Linda D'Agrosa, Maris Allen, Nancy Edison, Morgan and

Alonna Soderberg, Rose Wazana Benstock, Nancy Cassutt-Ison, Daryn Stier, Jillian Klarl, Betsy Allen, Ginger Hinchman-Birkeland, Caroline Douglas, Deirdre Mueller, Lee Smith, Marie Hartley, Laura Gill and Ella, Christine Ciavarella, Jeanine Martin, Kelsey Brendel, Eric Lieberman, Todd and Dixie Nelson, Marissa Nelson, Brad Pearsall, Lee Cook, Uma/Trish Schaef, Sally Smith, Cindy Olsen, Nathan Josephs, Kenny, Nikki, Jackie and Nicole Arends, Rene Parcell, Debra Benavidez, Sumant and Medini Pendharkar, Sudhanshu Kumar, Eirik Oeyo, Nina Liou, Lavonne Lewis, and Lorrie Caplan. To the mothers at Acta Technology who participated in interviews for this book, I want to thank: Joi Iwata-Yabumoto, Stephanie Ravizza, Shemaine Smith, Mary Jane Hagenau, and Sharon Han. You are all great mothers!

I extend a generous thank-you to Peter Workman for his generosity and savvy vision.

I have been privileged to call Ruth Sullivan my editor on several projects. Her talents always bring out the best in my writing. I hope we continue to work together. Thank you, Ruth.

*P*regnancy is one of the most profound passages in a woman's life. It is a time of reflection, inspiration, doubt, nervous anticipation, and awe. It is also a time to prepare: prepare for childbirth and the entry into motherhood. Shortly after conception, amazing changes take place within our body. Our breasts become tender, our tummy slowly swells, we often feel lethargic and spaced out. Next we can expect morning sickness, more fatigue, and then one day we can't fit into our favorite pair of jeans. The first time we hear our baby's heartbeat flutter like a bird's, we are moved to tears. The tiny being inside of us becomes more real with each passing day and we begin to ask ourselves all kinds of questions. "I wonder if it's a boy or a girl?" "Will he have dark hair and light eyes or the other way around?" "Will she enjoy traveling, skiing, or physics?" But we must wait, and wait some more, before these questions are finally answered.

As our belly expands into the world, and we experience our baby's movements, we are nudged by the miracle of life. We can hardly believe that we are creating this little being who tumbles inside of us, waiting to be released into our arms. We prepare our home for our newborn. Yet, more important, we prepare ourselves—making the inner adjustments necessary for bringing a child into the world. There are so many things to contend with, so many questions to answer, and so much to do. That is why I have written *Meditations During Pregnancy*. It can serve as a loving and supportive friend to help you navigate through this time of tremendous growth and change—emotionally and psychologically, as well as physically. *Meditations During Pregnancy* addresses the real-life concerns, the full range of emotions, conflicts, worries, and the day-to-day issues that arise during pregnancy.

Moreover, this book celebrates the journey into motherhood. May you find yourself among these pages and feel comforted by the fact that other women have come before you, and have experienced the very same things you are experiencing now. You are not alone in your feelings. The days of discomfort, the poetic side of pregnancy, the excitement and the fears are shared by all mothers, no matter where they find themselves on the globe. Welcome.

You can read the meditations straight through, at random, or use the topical index in the back to look up a particular concern.

A baby is God's opinion that the world should go on.
❦ CARL SANDBURG

Starting a family is an act of supreme optimism. And hope springs eternal in a mother's heart. When things go wrong, our hope for a better future carries us through. We believe in the gifts children offer the world, and we have faith in our ability to raise the next generation. We need to hold on to and nourish this belief, for it can make all the difference in the world, for us and for our children.

I will dream of a better tomorrow where the special gifts of children fill the future, and will work to build a world where those dreams can come true.

The pleasure of being a parent isn't reasonable or objective . . . it is the extraordinary experience of having short people who hang around a while, who can change you as they change, who push and prod and aggravate and thrill you and make life fuller. Who are, more than anything else, irrationally special to you.

ELLEN GOODMAN

*M*otherhood is good, bad, and everything in between. The joy of it doesn't always make sense. The reason we do it makes even less. Here we are, pregnant and expecting, on the verge of great change. Yet, even if we waited until the end of our childbearing years to decide to have a child, the reasons for our choice were ultimately probably not rational. No matter how many lists we made of the pros and cons of motherhood, no matter how much data we collected and analyzed, our final decision had more to do with faith and the desires of the human heart than reason.

I took a leap of faith when I decided to become a mother. My reasons don't have to make sense to others, only to me.

Oh who can tell the range of joy.
Or set the bounds of beauty?

🎵 SARA TEASDALE

here is nothing quite so delicious as having our beloved struck by one of Cupid's arrows. From out of nowhere, it seems, he is dumbfounded by our maternal radiance. Instead of perceiving us as rotund, in his eyes we have taken on the luminosity of Venus. He can't take his eyes off of us. We are the very picture of beauty. A masterpiece!

This is a rare and wonderful time in our life as a couple. It's great when we can both thoroughly enjoy it.

I feel as ripe as a melon, and as juicy.

🌸 MARGUERITE THOMAS

*P*regnancy can be an unexpected awaken-
ing. We suddenly feel voluptuous, sexy, fertile, and electric. The growth of our baby opens us
to our sensual nature, and we may feel aroused by
the simplest things: the way our partner straightens
his hair, bites into an apple, or brushes against us in
the kitchen. The freedom of not having to worry
about becoming pregnant is liberating and exciting.
We can explore our sexuality without fear of the
consequences. We can enjoy spontaneity and our
desire for ecstasy!

**I will open to my sensual self like a flower
meeting the rays of the sun.**

*God will only give you what he knows you can
handle.*

🐾 ANONYMOUS

*W*e wanted a baby, but this is ridiculous! For
years we hoped for a child and then we got
the news: twins (or even triplets) are on the way!
Already, we are panicking. We must buy twice
as much of everything: pacifiers, baby blankets,
booties, stroller, and cribs. Suddenly our house
doesn't seem big enough: the guest bedroom will
have to be transformed into a child's bedroom one
day, and from now on visitors will have to sleep on
the couch. And before we know it, we'll be thinking
about paying for two college educations! Prayers
are definitely in order.

**I prayed for a child and my prayers were more
than answered. Now I will pray for help.**

Anything worth doing is worth doing frantically.
♫ ANNE WILSON SCHAEF

*T*hose of us who do too much are so accustomed to doing everything in high gear that we often rush through our first pregnancy. We forget that pregnancy, like a fine wine, is to be savored and enjoyed. We can sit outside, basking in the spring sunshine. We can float on our backs in a pool, resting our hands on our tummy to feel the baby's movements. Why not walk along the beach or take a leisurely hike through the woods? Instead of folding our pregnancy into the frantic pace of our pre-parent lives, let's downshift and be present for this incredible experience.

I must slow down if I am to absorb and enjoy the novel experience of my first pregnancy.

In a child's lunchbox, a mother's thoughts.

❀ JAPANESE PROVERB

*D*uring all the excitement and confusion of pregnancy, it is important to remember that our other children can feel left out. They might feel that our special attention is going to the new baby, and fear that when he finally comes out, we won't love them anymore. While it is helpful to tell our children that even when they have a new brother or sister we won't stop loving them, the tiniest gestures of kindness can also help reassure them. Why not place a little note in his lunchbox or drop a little present in her pocket that she'll discover on her way to school? There are all kinds of simple ways to say, "I love you and I am thinking of you." Why not let them know now?

I will take extra measures to make sure my children know I love them as much as ever, even though I am wrapped up in my pregnancy. Little gestures of love go a long way.

You grow up the day you have your first real laugh at yourself.

ETHEL BARRYMORE

I remember interviewing a lovely expectant mother who, rather self-consciously, told me that some days she was so full of energy that she made a fool of herself. "I get these surges of energy, I don't know where they come from, but I feel like a frisky cat with spring fever," she said, her eyes lighting up mischievously. "My stomach is heavy, but I feel light."

Have you ever felt so happy you wanted to burst or shout out to the treetops? Expectant mothers often do. Expect it and enjoy it!

I will allow myself to act the fool and be giddy with delight.

My husband was so afraid we would never get to do any of the things we enjoyed once the baby was born that he bought tickets to plays, concerts and the symphony—all in the same month! I loved the performances even though I fell asleep through half of them.

♫ AMY REDDING

*I*t's easy to think that "life as we've known it" will all disappear once our baby is born. Although many aspects of our lives *will* change, that doesn't mean we have to completely give up adult activities forever.

If we haven't already done so, we should start looking for a trusted baby-sitter or a wonderful neighborhood grandmother who enjoys children. Then we can be assured of having plenty of chances to dress up and go out on the town, as adults, and feel confident that our baby is in competent hands.

I will find the help I need so my husband and I can continue to enjoy our favorite activities.

A baby's mother also needs a mother.

❧ ERICA JONG

*I*t doesn't matter whether we're pregnant with our first child or our fifth, we still need the support and guidance only a mother can provide. We need to talk to her about our hopes and frustrations; we need her to suggest helpful options to the questions that fill our heads; and we need her to give us a hug when we feel like we're the worst mother in the world.

While we must separate from our mother and become our own person, that doesn't mean we stop needing the kind of help that only a mother can give. If our own mother is no longer around, we need to remember what she taught us—and turn to other mothers for the advice and reassurance we need. Mothering is a big job—one of the biggest—and we need all the help we can get.

I am forever connected to my mother regardless of my age, level of maturity, or personal growth. Our bond is undeniable and invaluable.

There is nothing stronger in the world than gentleness.

🐾 HAN SUYIN

hose of us who have fought our way into the world of business, politics, or other male-dominated fields, have relied on our toughness and grit to get ahead. We learned that compassion and tenderness had to be left outside the office door. Although these tactics may have helped us to climb the corporate ladder, they are not the best ones for engaging in human relationships. Gentleness, patience, and understanding are better tools for the job of motherhood. If we're out of practice using these skills, we need not worry, because with a baby on the way we will get plenty of opportunities to polish them up again.

Gentleness is rarely valued in the work world. But at home, it will mean everything to my child.

All of my life I been like a doubled up fist . . . poundin', smashin', drivin'. Now I'm going to loosen these doubled up hands and touch things easy with them.
♫ TENNESSEE WILLIAMS

*H*ow many of us can relate to these words? We've spent so much time driving ourselves toward goals, we can't even remember the last time we relaxed. When we found out we were pregnant, one of our first reactions was to clench our teeth, determined not to let a baby slow us down.

If we're looking to give ourselves an early heart attack, we're well on our way. We cannot possibly stay uptight for so long and not bring injury to our body, mind, and spirit. Pregnancy is a great time to learn to let go of the Type A behaviors that might have brought us success in other endeavors—and *slow down.* One wise obstetrician tells his patients, "Don't stand when you can sit, and don't sit when you can lie down. And don't think when you rest you're 'doing nothing'—you're making a baby!"

I need to take steps to loosen my tight grasp on life. And the first thing I need to "touch easy" is myself.

It's imperative for both child and parents that the child be wanted.

🌸 MICHAEL COOKINGHAM

A wanted child is not the same as a planned one. While we may be surprised by a positive pregnancy test, and feel mixed emotions at the onset, we need to remember one thing: if a child is to feel wanted, we must welcome her with open arms. Otherwise, our ambivalence might be felt by the baby, and no matter how many material comforts we offer, a hole will remain in her heart.

The first and best thing I can do for my child is to genuinely want her as part of my family.

Babies are such a nice way to start people.
              DON HEROLD

*B*abies are special people. They gurgle and coo, their sweet-smelling skin reminiscent of fresh rose petals. They are soft to the touch and cute beyond belief, with miniature hands and toes. They look at us adoringly and their entire body wiggles with excitement whenever we enter a room. They remind us of what is good in the world.

I can hardly wait to be introduced to the special person inside of me.

Worry less, pray more.

♫ ANONYMOUS

*P*regnancy can be full of worries. We worry about straining our backs. We worry about taking sufficient amounts of vitamins and minerals and eating the right foods. If we are diabetic, we worry about our blood sugar levels and the strain on our kidneys. If we are anemic, we worry about getting enough iron. We even worry about whether worry is adversely affecting our baby!

Worry only wastes our energy. We must take whatever action is necessary to quell our fears and bring them into check. And then try not to worry.

Worry only compounds my concerns. Putting my energy toward finding a solution is time better spent.

I like being pregnant!

⚓ JANE HAGENEAU

*B*eing an expectant mother can feel like the most natural state in the world. We enjoy being round. We feel extremely feminine and sexy. We almost wish our pregnancy would never end so the good feelings continue.

Somehow, being pregnant pulls us into ourselves as though our tummies were a familiar universe for us to revel in. When we go out into the world, we carry this universe with us as though we have a delicious secret that everyone can see, yet no one can decipher. We feel the mystery within us and don't want to let it go.

I hope my pregnancy—or at least the feeling that goes with it—lasts well beyond nine months!

Nurturing Touch

Studies have shown that women who are touched in a nurturing way more easily transfer that nurturing to their babies.

🦶 PAULA KOEPKE

*H*uman beings need to be touched. However, many of us came from families where people were afraid of touch: they held back, rarely comforting us with physical strokes or caresses. Now that we are expectant mothers, we can break old patterns and start anew. We can learn about prenatal and sensual massage. We can let our hands reach out to others. We can trade back rubs with our partner to improve circulation and relax tensed-up muscles. Then, when our baby is born, we will feel more comfortable about massaging his little body, stroking his hair, outlining his eyebrows with our fingertips, and nourishing him with our sweet and generous touch.

Touch is a powerful way to connect with those I love. Just because my family of origin did not understand its value doesn't mean I have to follow in their footsteps.

When an infant is born, part of us dies.

♫ HELEN SMITH

Change always seems to be accompanied by loss. We give up a part of who we are in order to grow into a fuller, more mature self. Although the part of us that we give up is never completely gone, it will recede into the background, to be replaced by the new woman we are becoming. For some of us that means letting go of negative patterns holding us back. For others, change brings a renewed sense of our authentic selves, and we feel less self-conscious about expressing ourselves. One thing is certain—we are entering new territory, and we will inevitably grow.

Giving birth to my baby means giving birth to my new self. I will honor both of us as we enter a new world.

What is important to a relationship is a harmony of emotional roles. . . .

☙ MIRRA KOMAROVSKY

*P*regnancy is a good time to discuss the division of labor in our future household. Who will change the diapers, defrost the breast milk for night feedings, give our little one a bath and rock him to sleep? What if our infant has colic, chronic diaper rash, or croup? Which parent will be responsible for doctor's visits? Trips to the drugstore? Taking time off from work to relieve the nanny?

Baby's needs add up. That is why it is helpful to discuss our parental roles now, so we can have greater harmony later.

Being sensitive to each other's needs can greatly reduce the stresses involved in caring for a newborn. I would do well to discuss these issues with my husband *before* our baby is born.

The first duty of love is to listen.

🦶 Paul Tillich

istening is an art that requires focused attention not only with our ears but with our hearts as well. To truly listen to one another means we hear the feelings being shared as well as the words. We take in another's experience and attend to it with our entire being.

While it is always important to have friends who really hear us, it is especially important during pregnancy. We may have pressing questions and concerns that a true listener can help sort out. We may need reassurance and someone to share in our experience instead of giving us advice. That way, we will truly feel heard.

Listening is an act of love. I will gravitate to those friends who can be there for me during this special and sometimes overwhelming time, and will distance myself from those who can't.

Whatever you make of yourself, be sure of this—that you are dreadfully like other people.

♪JAMES RUSSELL LOWELL

*W*hen we first become pregnant we feel elated, expectant with bliss. The poetic side of pregnancy is all we can see. Becoming a mother is all we can think about. "I'll never get morning sickness," we tell ourselves. "I couldn't possibly gain more than twenty-five pounds," we smugly assert. Then it hits—morning sickness, weight gain, fatigue—and we ruefully discover how much we have in common with all the other pregnant women of the world.

I will join the universal clan of expectant mothers for better or worse, in sickness and in health.

Did it hurt when you fell from heaven?

🌸 JASON PASCHIS

*R*emember how it felt when you first fell in love? The feelings were so pure and tender. You gazed upon your beloved and your heart was filled with the sweetness—and oblivious to any bad habits or annoying traits. In your eyes, he was perfect.

One of the greatest joys of having a baby is being filled with these same feelings all over again. The perfection of a newborn's tiny fingers and the small of his neck awakens the most innocent kind of love in our hearts, and when we gaze into our little one's eyes, we see that love returned. Our baby is fresh from heaven.

I await my baby's birth as proof that there is, indeed, perfection in the world. To me, she is heaven sent.

Let me put this as gently as I know how: parenthood is a state from which you never recover.

🦶 JULIE TILSNER

Someone once said: "If people really knew what they were getting into once they had kids, they'd never have them." The truth is, parenthood changes everything. Life is never the same. *We* are never the same. Our children bend and shape us as much as we shape them. Their interests are not necessarily our interests. Our favorite things to do are not necessarily their favorite things to do. As in a marriage, we must expand and work around each other's needs while keeping in touch with our own. And realize that no matter how much we might resist, we are going to change.

If parenthood changes me for the better, I may not want to fully recover.

*How might your life have been different if there had
been a place for you? A place for you to go . . . a place
of women, to help you learn the ways of woman . . . a
place where you were nurtured from an ancient flow
sustaining you and steadying you . . .*

♫ JUDITH DUERK

hildbirth is an incredible passage. And like
other rites of passage it should come with
support and celebration. What if we were to gather
together our closest women friends and invent our
own ritual? We'd form a circle of strength to sustain
us as we embark on the timeless journey into motherhood. We would open the circle to grandmothers
and aunts who could share their wisdom, talking to
us about our hopes and fears, what it means to be a
mother, what we will give up and what we will
gain.

What if we created a sacred place that sustains us
as we cross over into the realm of motherhood? A
place where we belong. A place where the wisdom
of the mothers is passed on.

**I can create a circle of support and celebration
with the many women in my life. There will be a
place for me.**

Fate chooses our relatives, we choose our friends.
🌸 JACQUES DELILLE

*C*ertain friends make a pregnancy even more special. They gladly share every detail and new development with us: the first heartbeat, the results of the sonogram, the choosing of Baby's name. They throw a baby shower and give such a thoughtful gift, it brings tears to our eyes. When our baby arrives, they are the first ones to greet us at the hospital. Having them makes the events of our lives seem more poignant *and* more real.

I am lucky to have such special friends. Life wouldn't be the same without them.

Hope is not the conviction that something will turn out well but the certainty that something makes sense, regardless of how it turns out.

VACLAV HAVEL

*P*regnancy, for some of us, is not initially a welcomed blessing. We're not sure about the man we're with; our parents think we're too young; we haven't completed our studies; and our savings account is not as robust as we'd like. The fact is, we might choose not to marry the father. We may need to ask for some financial assistance from family and friends—and we might have to take on adult responsibilities sooner than we had planned. Yet, amid all the potential negatives, we hold the faith deep within us that the future will be bright.

Now is the time when I must have faith in myself. My roots are strong; they keep the light.

If a man does not keep pace with his companions, perhaps it is because he hears a different drummer. Let him step to the music which he hears, however measured or far away.

♪ HENRY DAVID THOREAU

Not all expectant mothers are alike. Some of us want to be knocked out during labor while others want to sit in a hot tub and deliver a baby underwater. Some of us are working with doctors, others with midwives. Some of us look forward eagerly to the experience of breast-feeding, others dread it. Rather than judge each other, why not be open to the differences among us? This will come in handy when, as parents, we are forced to deal effectively with other parents whose philosophies, practices, and beliefs are very different from our own.

There are many ways to birth a baby. I will decide which way is best for me and my child—and will try not to second-guess my decisions.

Infants whose mothers exercised regularly through their pregnancy seem to be more neurodevelopmentally advanced.

🌸 TRACY TEARE

The benefits of exercise during pregnancy are broad ranging. Our muscles stay toned. We work out stress, tension, and aggression. We feel good about ourselves. And we like the way we look. But do we know about the benefits to our developing child as well?

According to recent studies, a mother's exercise during pregnancy helps to develop the infant's nervous system. In fact, a study from Case Western Reserve University claims, "At five days old, these babies were significantly better at quieting themselves when exposed to stimuli than infants born to inactive mothers." So, if we haven't been doing a weekly exercise routine, we might want to start one now.

Exercise maintains my health and gives my baby a better start in life.

My husband and I decided it would be best if he stayed home with the kids since my job was more flexible and higher paying.

🦶 KATHLEEN JORDAN

While it's not as unusual as it would have been in the 1950s, having a husband who stays home with the kids is still not the norm. Some family members, not completely comfortable with the arrangement, may ask when he will be returning to work. Neighbors might stare or shake their heads in disapproval. Hopefully, our family and friends will understand and will let us know we have their support. "I know this is the best arrangement for your child," they'll tell us. Or "What a lucky kid to have a father who is so involved!" And they'll be right!

It takes courage to go against the norm. Fortunately, my husband and I don't mind being pioneers, especially when it is in the best interest of our child.

*In all things of nature there is something of the
marvelous.*

♫ ARISTOTLE

*L*et's face it, not every day of pregnancy is
awe-inspiring—some days are purely awful.
We're overly emotional and take offense at the most
ridiculous things. We feel fat, tired, and swollen.
Our temper flares. Tears soak our pillow. We complain and wonder why we put ourselves through
this.

If we can remember that these days will pass,
then we will be better able to get through them,
knowing that those happier aspects will surface
once again.

**Pregnancy is indeed marvelous. It just may not
be marvelous every single day.**

— Trouble: Seeing the Humor in It —

My mother had trouble with me, but I think she enjoyed it.

❧ MARK TWAIN

t starts in the womb, with them pushing their little heads into our bladder, creating real discomfort. Then a friend comes along, sees the agonized look on our face, and makes us laugh so hard we have to dash to the nearest rest room. At the symphony, we expect our little one to rest quietly through the solo violin, when suddenly, he taps his little feet so vigorously that the person next to us stares at all the activity beneath our dress!

It starts before they are born—the comical antics. But the kind of trouble babies create just makes us laugh.

Undoubtedly, my child will give me trouble. Hopefully, I will see the humor in it.

A smiling face is half the meal.

LATVIAN PROVERB

Nothing brings a smile to a pregnant woman's face faster than coming home from work to find her husband at the stove cooking. While the smell of dinner wafts in from the other room, she can put up her feet, thumb through a magazine, or read a letter from an old friend.

No, nothing brings a smile to a pregnant woman's face like the sight of her husband making dinner for two. Unless, of course, he's doing it in the nude!

My glowing smile of thanks will be reward enough for my husband's generous efforts.

One of the most exciting observations of our era is the discovery that the newborn has the ability to find his mother's breast all on his own and decide for himself when to take his first feeding.

♫ MARSHALL AND PHYLLIS KLAUS

Newborns are amazing! They're born knowing how and when to feed and in our arms instinctively position their heads to suckle from our breast. Straight from the womb they recognize the beat of our heart. If their freshly birthed body is laid on top of our belly immediately after delivery, they will not cry unless removed. And, at less than thirty minutes old, they can tell the difference between their mother and a blanketed bassinet—and their preference is for us, *mother.*

My infant will come into the world knowing me like no other.

*Keep in mind that no matter what your personal
qualifications for motherhood happen to be, you can
be sure that you will surprise yourself by being quite
fit to deal with some of the situations you were wor-
ried about. And you will be less prepared than you
imagined for certain others.*

⚓ HARRIET LERNER

*E*xpectant mothers beware! You are about to
embark on a journey that will stretch you in
ways you can't imagine, challenge your strongest
beliefs, test your limits on a daily basis, and make
you a better person whether you like it or not. Becoming a mother is an act of ultimate courage. You
will be tested, tried, and judged, often most harshly
by yourself. You will increase your power and wisdom, and you will learn how to be more human
and humane. You will make dreadful mistakes and
experience incredible victories.

Whether you know it or not, you have enlisted in
one of the toughest campaigns known to humankind. Arm yourself.

**Motherhood is the ultimate boot camp. I will
prepare for its daily rigors and keep in mind that
when things get tough, the tough don't stop, they
just roll up their sleeves and attack!**

Self-pity is our worst enemy, and if we yield to it, we can never do anything wise in this world.

🦶 HELEN KELLER

*P*regnancy is supposed to be a happy time, but what if we are depressed by our current circumstances? What if we had never imagined this would be the way things would turn out? What if we feel disappointed by the size of our home or the fact that we still live in a one-bedroom apartment? If we view our lives through the lens of self-pity, we may be cursing ourselves for becoming pregnant "at a time like this."

But the truth is, there is never a perfect time. And while we can work on improving our lives, it is good to remember that, to our little one, we will still be "the best mommy on earth" no matter what our circumstances. Children don't need big homes or lots of fancy clothing—but they do need happy parents.

Self-pity is self-defeating. I will have the courage to "change the things I can, accept the things I cannot change, and pray for the wisdom to know the difference."

Is not a young mother one of the sweetest sights life shows us?

♪ WILLIAM MAKEPEACE THACKERY

$\mathcal{M}$anufactured images of beauty bombard us on billboards, magazine covers, and television advertisements. And while some cultures celebrate the full, round, pregnant body, unfortunately ours does not.

There's no escaping the culture we live in. And while we all wish to look our best, we must keep in mind that our best may not look the same as the images around us. In fact, chances are, most of us will *never* look much like the commercial images, since the average model now weighs 23 percent less than the average woman!

Pregnancy is not an appropriate time to diet. It is, however, an excellent time to eat more healthfully, exercise frequently (with our doctor's approval), and engage in activities that reduce stress: yoga, massage, and Pilates. We will not only feel better, but we will look better, too.

I will take good care of my body during pregnancy—a long-term investment in my own health and beauty.

_We are ourselves creations . . . and we, in turn,
are meant to continue creativity, by being creative
ourselves._

❦ JULIA CAMERON

Gestation is one of the most potent forms of
creativity. It often sparks the creative fire
within us and we find ourselves wanting to learn to
play the guitar, dust off the paintbrushes in our
closet, remodel the bathroom or kitchen, put bows
in the dog's hair, or introduce a new product to the
CEO! Our waking life is full of possibility. Our
dreams are vivid. The Muse is calling and we hear
our names in the wind.

**It doesn't matter how I express my creativity as
long as I express it. I am full of creation.**

Babe Ruth struck out 1,330 times.

👣 ANONYMOUS

*W*hen we're feeling disgruntled, we all have a tendency to compare our insides with others' outsides. We focus on their successes, forgetting the times they, too, have struck out. "Her pregnancies always go so easily," we complain. "She never gains any weight," we mumble under our breath. "Her husband always helps out." But the fact is, we don't know exactly what it's like to be in the other person's shoes. For all we know, those expectant mothers who seem to be so carefree and to "have it all together" might actually be jealous of us!

It is futile to compare myself with others. Everyone strikes out sometimes. I just may not see it. I have to focus on *my* life because it's the only one I can really know.

*Practice sidling up to open windows without being
detected. Stay away from quiet environments. Learn
some good farting jokes.*

♪JENNIFER LOUDEN

*F*latulence is one of the more embarrassing
aspects of pregnancy. If you have tried changing your diet, getting more exercise, and doing yoga
without satisfactory results, you might just have to
grin and bear it.

A sense of humor during pregnancy is not only
useful, it's essential. Because, the truth is, some
aspects of pregnancy are far from glamorous. When
we burp and fart like sailors, it's difficult to think of
ourselves as "delicate flowers." So we can explore
another side of ourselves—and learn to laugh
about it.

**I will handle my sometimes unruly bodily
expressions with humor and, whenever possible,
with an air of sophistication.**

I was so inexperienced as to think that having a baby was a perfectly natural process.

🌺 ISADORA DUNCAN

*I*n most parts of the world, pregnancy and childbirth is a natural process woven into the fabric of daily life. But here in the United States we have many options about childbirth as well as medical requirements. As a result, we must educate ourselves. Do we want a home birth? Do we want a water birth? Will insurance cover alternative methods? Would we prefer delivering the baby in a hospital? Under what conditions is a C-section likely? What percentage of the time does our obstetrician deliver vaginally, and how often does she perform a C-section? It's a nine-month crash course. Better get out our pencils and notebooks. Class is in session.

Educating myself about pregnancy and childbirth will help me feel more confident when the real test is at hand.

*It sometimes happens, even in the best of families,
that a baby is born. This is not necessarily a cause
for alarm. The important thing is to keep your wits
about you and borrow some money.*

👣 ELINOR GOULDING SMITH

Not all relatives are child-friendly. They view
children with a skeptical eye and loathe
the messes they make. They do not find insects
interesting, nor do they enjoy being asked the same
question a dozen times. They expect children,
including infants, to be seen and not heard.

With relatives like these, the best thing to do is be
prepared. If our baby bangs her spoon on the high
chair tray, splattering Thanksgiving gravy on the
guests, we can move in quickly with moist towel-
ettes. If she spits out an unsavory morsel, all we
have to do is hide it under her mountain of peas.
Or, should she grab a hank of Auntie's hair, we
should smile, remove the little hand, and pass on as
though nothing happened.

**Children and faux pas go together. I will not
allow the disapproving looks of relatives make
me or my child feel ashamed of her behavior.**

Having a baby is like suddenly getting the world's worst roommate, like have Janis Joplin with a bad hangover and PMS come to stay with you.

♪ANNE LAMOTT

*L*ike an unruly live-in, a baby can turn our lives upside down. They're demanding, they keep late hours, and they certainly don't clean up after themselves. Their moods change every other minute, they run up the bills without offering to pay their share, and they don't give us a moment's privacy. Why, then, do we do it? Is it simply some genetic impulse to perpetuate the human race? Of course not. Once you've had a baby, you'll know!

Having a baby is part of the absurd logic of the human heart. If only they came with operating instructions.

Food is an important part of a balanced diet.
❀ FRAN LEBOWITZ

*P*regnancy is not the time to start dieting or skipping meals. Our growing baby is absorbing every nutrient available. If we do not replenish all the iron, folic acid, calcium, and other vitamins and minerals our baby is using, there won't be any left for our own body. So, if we are accustomed to dieting to keep svelte when we're without child, we must think again now that we are eating for two.

I will eat regular meals during my pregnancy to keep myself—and my baby—healthy and strong.

Wow! You're action-packed!

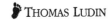 THOMAS LUDIN

*I*sn't it wonderful to see our older children welcome our baby home? "He smells nice," they tell us after putting their nose on top of the baby's head. Or, "He stinks," after Baby has filled his pants. When they see him wiggle with delight as his beloved siblings enter the room, they are astounded. They thought a baby would just be a big lump and lay there. Instead, he's action-packed.

My children will be delighted with the novelty of their new brother or sister.

Natural Childbirth

*I was first startled, and then pleased, that someone
had ranked natural childbirth on the same level as
killing a grizzly bear. . . . I, who was always the wimp
in gym class whom nobody wanted on their team,
felt vindicated.*

♪ JENNIFER, IN *LABOR DAY*

hildbirth can be empowering. We experience a level of physical intensity that may not
have been part of our previous life experience. Our
self-image may have been one of a wimp: someone
who possessed a low threshold, or no tolerance, for
pain. But natural childbirth can change all that.
Once we have withstood hours of labor without the
use of medication, we may believe, like Jennifer,
that from now on we "can do anything."

**Childbirth without painkillers can make me feel
less like a wimp—and more like Xena the
Warrior Princess.**

Success is a science. If you have the conditions, you get the results.

🌸 OSCAR WILDE

Some of us have tried to get pregnant for years. We have gone through surgeries, had eggs extracted and implanted, hoped and prayed that our body wouldn't reject the fetus; then one day, it happens. We are verifiably pregnant and, as the doctor says, "everything looks good!" At first we might feel tentative, unsure whether the baby is here to stay. But as the pregnancy progresses and we receive high marks during our exams, we may feel ecstatic and even a little cocky. We dance around the house strutting, then raise our fist in triumph: "Yes!"

There's nothing like sweet success.

Experience is the name everyone gives to their mistakes.

🦶 DOROTHY PARKER

*E*veryone makes mistakes. CEOs miscalculate the success of a product, counselors occasionally give bad advice, and bus drivers make wrong turns. However, if we learn from our mistakes they'll become part of a valuable experience from which we grow.

As expectant mothers we should get used to the fact that we're going to make mistakes. We might gain too much weight or eat the wrong foods. In our general expansiveness during pregnancy, we often buy too much only to discover that our child won't use some items until she's in kindergarten! Whatever our mistakes, we need not berate ourselves—just chalk them up to good experience.

Mistakes are how I learn new ways of doing things.

Having a baby can feel like winning the lottery, getting everything you wanted for Christmas, and falling in love all wrapped into one. It can also feel like being marooned on a deserted arctic island in a blizzard, naked, with only Rush Limbaugh for company.

♫ JENNIFER LOUDEN

*M*ixed emotions come with the territory of "Pregnancy" and "Motherhood." If we've never experienced them before, we will now. Elation, euphoria, bliss, awe . . . But also loneliness, fear, confusion, resentment. My friend Betsy, who became a mother at forty, confided: "I've experienced different emotions, but they usually come a few minutes apart. Now they all come at once!"

Certainly, these contradictory emotional states can be overwhelming. Yet, if we know about them, we will not be so dumbfounded when they first hit us. Eventually we will come to terms with the fact that "mixed emotions" are just part of being a mom.

Living in the land of emotional extremes is the stuff motherhood is made of. I will learn to come to terms with this fact and just keep doing the best I can, no matter how I feel at any given moment.

No man walks out of the delivery room the same man who walked in.

⚓ JAMES DOUGLAS BARRON

*W*hile the focus of attention is usually on the mother during pregnancy and birth, it is important to remember that our husbands are experiencing incredible changes as well. They may not be particularly forthcoming when it comes to verbalizing their feelings, so we may see strange alterations in their behavior until we understand more about what they're going through.

Just being quiet doing the dishes together or putting on a favorite album that helps him to unwind can open the door to intimate conversation. Or why not just ask him how he thinks the baby will affect him? Even if he answers with a typical male shrug, he'll probably be secretly pleased that you cared enough to ask.

Talking about the changes my husband and I are facing will strengthen our communication— something we'll need desperately in the months to come.

I saw pure love when my son looked at me, and I knew I had to make a good life for the two of us. . . .
SUZANNE SOMERS

here is nothing like the look of love in a newborn's eyes: love without reservation; love without condition. And complete and total trust. It will spark something inside that will mature us instantly. No longer will we be solely responsible for ourselves. We will be responsible for an innocent being who depends on us for his every need. All I will need to create a good life for my baby is to look in his eyes and see how much he needs me.

To be truly committed to another, my commitment must rest on pure love.

The best part of pregnancy for me? Honestly, I'd have to say the wet dreams. My doctor stiffly referred to them as "nocturnal orgasms." Either way, I loved them. Best sex I ever had!

♫ MARIA SANDOVAL

*I*t's true. Pregnancy may be the first time some of us have experienced spontaneous orgasms in our sleep. It's a pleasant surprise. We cry out in ecstasy, inadvertently waking our husband, who assumes, of course, that we are having a bad dream. Although he may try to comfort us with the best of intentions, he'd be smarter to just jump right in and join the fun.

Hot, sexy dreams are common for expectant mothers. I will enjoy them to the fullest.

At work, you think of the children you've left at home. At home, you think of the work you've left unfinished. Such a struggle is unleashed within yourself: your heart is rent.

❧ GOLDA MEIR

While some of us are perfectly happy to stay home with our children, others are not. Perhaps we have careers that do not lend themselves to extended time off. Maybe we know ourselves well enough to realize that the daily demands of being a stay-at-home mom are not for us. Some of us love our work so much that we can't imagine giving it up for our children. Others don't have the option of staying home: We need the income.

Working mothers are, by definition, divided souls. We constantly juggle the demands of our work and the needs of our children, knowing that we will never get it right every time. And that's okay.

I will take the responsibility of parenthood seriously, realizing that as a working mother, I will sometimes have to choose between professional obligations and family ones.

If I knew what I was anxious about, I wouldn't be so anxious.

MIGNON MCLAUGHLIN

Sometimes our fears and anxieties about the changes we're about to undergo, and the new responsibilities we're taking on, manifest themselves in funny ways. A friend of mine who went through years of infertility treatments tells me that when she was finally pregnant, she had a recurring nightmare that she would forget to pick up her child from daycare. Another mother dreamed that she was constantly late for final exams, but no matter how hard she searched, she could never find the classroom.

Whatever inadequacies we may fear, we must reassure ourselves that, when the time comes, we will be able to gather all the resources we need to meet this new and demanding role. When our overactive subconscious suggests otherwise, we can learn to laugh it off and remember it was only a dream.

I will use my dreams to help me discover the secret fears I need to confront as I face the biggest responsibility of my life.

It is the ability to choose which makes us human.
♪ MADELEINE L'ENGLE

We've all heard about the benefits of breast-feeding. However, some of us are not sure we want to become involved in such an all-consuming venture. Perhaps our work schedule prevents us from pumping milk between board meetings. Maybe our husband wants to play a more active role by handling those middle-of-the-night feedings. Or, after hearing about painful breast infections and cracked nipples, we're not sure we want to endure such an ordeal.

There's no need to decide now whether or not we will nurse our baby. When the time comes we can try it and see how it goes, and ask for help if we need it. Then we can begin to choose what is best for us, our baby, and our lifestyle.

The choice to breast-feed is mine. I expect others to respect my decision, whatever it may be.

Raising children is far more creative than most jobs for men and women.

⚘ BENJAMIN SPOCK

*I*t's wonderful that we live in a time when so many options are available to mothers. However, those of us who choose to be stay-at-home mothers sometimes feel like we're being judged. Others treat us as if we're not smart enough or ambitious enough to do anything else.

It's a sad fact that mothers' work is still considered less valuable than other forms of labor. We might need to remind others as tactfully and clearly as we can, that taking care of children is important, inspiring, challenging, and demanding work. To do it well requires every bit as much intelligence, creativity, problem-solving, and management ability as the more prestigious, high-paying jobs. And those of us who choose to make child rearing our full-time pursuit, whether for a few months or the rest of our lives, deserve as much respect as those of us in the paid labor force.

If I choose to stay at home with my child I will expect others to respect my decision and support me. We may structure our lives differently, but in the end, we are all mothers.

In general, my children refused to eat anything that hadn't danced on TV.

👣 ERMA BOMBECK

$\mathcal{T}$rying to get older siblings to eat the vitamin-charged meals we are ingesting during pregnancy is no easy trick. More than likely, they prefer sugar-coated cereals, frozen waffles, spaghetti, and prepackaged lunches loaded with processed cheese and candy for dessert. So they may not mind the fact that we are microwaving more frozen dinners than usual, popping Pop-Tarts in the toaster, and dumping boxes of macaroni and cheese into boiling water. The fact is, we don't want to have to cook every meal twice.

While I'm pregnant I will do my best to prepare nutritious meals that everyone can enjoy, but I may have to rely on convenience foods more often until the baby is born.

What are the three words guaranteed to humiliate men everywhere? "Hold my purse."

♫ SANDRA BULLOCK

*R*eal men don't eat quiche, they don't ask for directions, and they wouldn't be caught dead holding a woman's purse. For those of us with husbands who are easily humiliated by carting around unmasculine objects, we'd better prepare them for the upcoming identity crisis. Not only might they be asked to hold our handbag so we can manage the baby, but they will be loaded up with a diaper bag, baby blankets, a stroller, and stuffed animals. As for the interior of their car (the last male bastion), it may become littered with teething biscuits, pacifiers, and sunshades that read: "Baby on Board." Yes, we'd better reassure them that real men carry a briefcase, a tool belt, *and* baby's belongings.

I will let my husband know that I think he is more of a man, not less of one, for helping me tote Baby's belongings around.

Pregnancy permits a woman to rationalize performances which otherwise would appear absurd.
❧ HELENE DEUTSCH

*P*regnancy lets us get away with things we wouldn't even attempt under normal circumstances. If we don't like Aunt Edna's pot roast, we can feign a sick stomach and pick up a pizza on the way home. If annoying neighbors invite themselves over, we can tell them we're exhausted and plan to retire early. Why wait in line for the public toilet when we can walk to the front of the queue and ask to use the next available stall? And watch us rationalize to a police officer that we can barely reach the pedals now that we've adjusted the seat to accommodate our belly.

My performances will be many during pregnancy. Hopefully, they'll be memorable.

I had an inestimable desire to eat apples. I have never liked them before.

🦶 ANNE BOLEYN

No one knows why pregnant women have such unusual cravings, but we do. Foods we didn't even like previously, we now can't get enough of. By the same token, foods we've always enjoyed may now repulse us. Certain smells wafting from the kitchen can cause nausea, while others make us ravenous. There is no rhyme or reason for it. It is just one of the many quirks of pregnancy.

It doesn't matter what foods I crave, as long as they are healthy and I eat them in moderation.

If I am not for myself, who will be for me? If I am only for myself, what am I? And if not now, when?

🎵 RABBI HILLEL

*R*emember that exercise class we promised ourselves we'd sign up for at the beginning of the year? Why haven't we done it? And what about the night-school class on promoting our business? Why haven't we taken it yet?

While preparing for the baby consumes a great deal of our time, it should not be used as yet another excuse to procrastinate, to avoid doing the things we know are important. As the saying goes, "There's no time like the present."

Now is the time to complete projects, tie up loose ends, and do things that will not be so easy to do once the baby's here. (Hint: Getting back to them will most likely take longer than you can imagine. Really.)

There is nothing on earth like the moment of seeing one's first baby . . . there is no height like this simple one. . . .

❧ KATHARINE TREVELYAN

Seeing our first child is unlike any other experience on earth. Everything is so new, so fresh. We gaze upon our child and, to us, she looks perfect. "She's the most beautiful baby in the world," we say to our midwife. "She's amazing!" Although midwives have heard these very same things before, they understand. After all, for us, it's a first.

When I take my first look, my heart will skip a beat.

The Luxury of Sleep

People who say they sleep like a baby usually don't have one.

🦶 LEO BURKE

*R*arely do babies sleep through the night. Instead, they wake up every few hours crying for food. That is why seasoned mothers encourage first-time expectant moms to sleep in on the weekends, snuggle up for a midafternoon nap, and excuse themselves early from evening engagements so they don't stay out too late. When our baby comes home, sleep may be a luxury we can no longer afford.

During my pregnancy, I will take every opportunity to sleep without interruption. I want to be well rested for the big arrival.

*No one understands how someone so little can so
change their world—until they hold their baby in
their arms.*

♫ PAM BROWN

*E*veryone tells us how much our world will
be turned upside down once Baby arrives.
"You'll never get any sleep," they tell us. "You'll be
lucky if you get to shower before noon," they warn.
"You're not going to be able to accomplish anything
around the house." While we smile politely and
nod, the truth is, we're skeptical of their ranting. "I
know life will change," we say to ourselves, "but it
can't change that much." Just wait. It can.

**Until I hold my baby in my arms I may not fully
comprehend the profound changes my child will
bring.**

You have to ask children and birds how cherries and strawberries taste.
🌸 JOHANN WOLFGANG VON GOETHE

*P*regnancy has a tendency to heighten our senses. Strawberries taste sweeter, and melons and papayas delight our taste buds. When we take a sip of wine, every nuance of flavor bursts in our mouth. We bury our noses in a bouquet, inhaling a multitude of exquisite fragrances. The smell of hot pretzels is irresistible; our husband's aftershave makes our heart palpitate; a wet kiss leaves our entire body tingling, hungry for more.

My heightened senses put the "extra" into ordinary.

Through a child's eyes we rediscover the world's loveliness and mystery.

👣 PAM BROWN

It is easy for adults to become focused on the leaves that need to be raked in the yard, the dishes that need to be washed, and the bills that need to be paid. Yet, if we can take a moment to see the world as our child sees it, we might be surprised. A pile of dead leaves is a playground of fun. Dirty dishes? Just an excuse to splash around in warm, bubbly water. With a little child's imagination the most mundane things can be transformed.

Today I will change my lens and try to see the world as if through the eyes of a child.

The reward of labor is life.

♪ WILLIAM MORRIS

hen we think of labor, we most often think of the actual birthing process. But the fact is, motherhood is comprised of different facets of labor. While we are pregnant our body works hard to create a fully formed infant. Then, in the delivery room, we toil and sweat and cry tears of joy once our baby is released from the womb. From that day forward we will offer our guidance, love, and wisdom, laboring to rear a child who is happy, healthy, and fulfilled.

My hard work will be rewarded with a beautiful new life.

It was tempting to think that if only they could speak, infants could take us back to their beginnings, to the force of their becoming; they could tell us about patience, about waiting and waiting in the dark.

JANE HAMILTON

Pregnancy takes patience. As much as we might want to expedite the process, there is nothing we can do to move it along. It takes nine months to make a baby, and like it or not, we must wait until the nine months are up before our infant is finally placed in our arms. At times it might seem like an endless waiting game, and we are eager to witness the results. Yet we must allow the force of our baby's becoming to unfold in its own time.

Whether I am waiting in line, waiting to turn the corner, or waiting to deliver my baby, patience is involved. I will do my best not to "rush through" my pregnancy.

*Being pregnant is like carrying a secret with
you wherever you go. You always know the baby
is there even if those around you are oblivious of his
presence.*

🦶 PAGE EDMUNDS

"*A*re you always aware of your baby being
inside of you?" one pregnant woman was
asked. Her reply: "Absolutely." Being pregnant is
like sharing a secret. Regardless of the situation,
we're always privy to the life within us. It doesn't
matter if we're speaking to the gas station attendant,
waiting in line at the bank, or sitting on a crowded
plane, our baby is never far from our thoughts.

**My baby and I share an intimate secret. It
belongs to both of us.**

Your mother loves you like the deuce while you are coming. Wrapped up here under her heart is perhaps the coziest time in existence. Then she and you are one, companions.

♫ EMILY CARR

ate in our pregnancy we can identify tiny baby parts as they form outlines on our bellies from within. It may be the first time we've truly been able to believe that an actual person is inside of us. And we want to meet this little person, to cradle him in our arms. We are eager to look into his eyes and cuddle him at the breast, wrapped in the intimacy of love.

But we should savor the wonderful coziness of pregnancy, and enjoy every minute of it. Never again will we be so close in quite the same way. Never again will caring for and protecting our child be so easy.

I will wait for my child with loving anticipation, holding on to the joy of pregnancy until the time for birth is here.

Music produces a kind of pleasure which human nature cannot do without.

⚘ CONFUCIUS

*M*ore and more studies illustrate the importance of music to a developing fetus. Not only does music have a calming effect on the baby, resulting in fewer kicks in the womb, but it is believed to help stimulate brain development. Don Campbell, author of *The Mozart Effect*, tells the story of Boris Brott, conductor of the Hamilton Philharmonic Orchestra in Ontario. Evidently, "Mr. Brott was puzzled by the fact that he could play some music by ear while he had to labor to master most pieces. He later learned from his mother that she had played the selections that came to him effortlessly while pregnant."

Whether we play music to increase our baby's intelligence or to bring joy to both of us, one thing is certain: music is a pleasure we cannot live without.

I will listen to my most cherished pieces of music with my growing baby whenever I can. It's a way of learning "by heart."

A Mother's Voice

He could fiddle all the bugs off a sweet-potato vine.
STEPHEN VINCENT BENÉT

Whether we hum to the stereo, sound out each note as we plunk out a tune on the piano, or sing our favorite songs, our voice carries sweet melodies to our little one's ears. Serving as a sonic umbilical, our voice soothes our baby with lullabies and folk tunes, rounds and magical sounds. It keeps rhythm with the beating of our heart, the movement of our digestion, and the ebb and flow of air moving in and out of our lungs. And once our infant is fresh from the womb, it is our voice that will greet him first and continue to enrich his world.

My voice will serve as the instrument of my love. May I play it sweetly.

I was so eager to know the sex of my child, I could hardly stand it. But my husband decided that he'd rather wait. I spent three agonizing months trying not to reveal this incredible secret.

♫ HELENA ELFMAN

t takes tremendous restraint to keep a secret. When the secret is the sex of our baby, it's almost impossible. Conversations about the baby must be kept gender-neutral. We can't discuss scenarios of "life with baby" that might give away the secret or exclaim, "Oh, I can just see you and our little boy out in the yard playing catch!"

If our husband wants to be surprised, we might be better off not knowing ourselves.

Secrets are hard to keep. It might be easier on my marriage if my doctor is the only one who knows whether it's a boy or a girl before the birth.

Humour . . . exaggerates the anxieties and absurdities we feel, so that we gain distance and, through laughter, relief.

        ❧ SARA DAVIDSON

*E*ver notice how much nervous laughter reverberates around the room of a natural-birthing class? And it's no wonder. Our instructor wastes no time getting into the nitty-gritty of the birthing process. She discusses the female anatomy in the most graphic terms and inundates us with information about all the things that can go wrong. Why, some of the words she regularly uses are the same ones our parents forbade us to say in their house!

The result: lots of laughter. But that's okay: laughter helps us to become more comfortable with the normal anxieties involved with becoming first-time parents.

Really, when you think about it, lots of things about the whole business of birth are a bit ridiculous!

The greatest battle that was ever fought—
Shall I tell you where and when?
On the maps of the world you will find it not;
It was fought by the mothers of men.

👣 JOAQUIN MILLER

Some of us will, for the first time in our life, find ourselves stepping up to the plate when it comes to taking care of our new baby—even when she has not yet wiggled out of the womb. We find we are becoming less intimidated by bossy nurses or patronizing obstetricians. If we don't get our questions answered adequately the first time, we persist until we can determine what is the best choice for our baby. We probe for more information even when professionals brush us off by suggesting we read yet another book on pregnancy. We won't take no for an answer when we ask to have our newborn brought to us for a middle-of-the-night feeding. We will start standing up for our wee one now, and we will never stop.

I will fight for what is best for my child, even if that means sticking my neck out and, occasionally, annoying the powers that be.

A request not to worry is perhaps the least soothing message capable of human utterance.

♫ MIGNON G. EBERHART

*P*regnancy and worry go together. So many things could go wrong! While we eat healthy meals, exercise, take prenatal vitamins, and follow doctor's orders, we can't help but wonder how we'd react if there was something wrong with the baby. If we have specific concerns, we should address them with our doctor or midwife during our next visit—or call them on the phone if our question can't wait. There's no such thing as a silly question, and chances are, they've heard them all before and are more than happy to help us through moments like these. Sometimes, simply verbalizing our worries can help allay them. We can also share our concerns with friends who have children (remember, they've been here, too!).

I will take the best possible care of my baby and myself during pregnancy; then I will learn to put worry aside and get on with what I have to do.

The world is wide, and I will not waste my life in friction when it could be turned into momentum.

⚜ FRANCES WILLARD

*A*dding a baby to a marriage can put terrible strain on the relationship. And for a time, points of conflict can be amplified. The fact is, this is a highly stressful period in which two lives are turned upside down, while a third is struggling to get started. It isn't easy to handle all the new situations that are about to be thrown at us by a little cyclone of energy.

Eventually, of course, there is much to bring husband and wife back together in their new incarnation as parents. But in the meantime, it can be rough. The more the two of us can plan now, before the baby comes, the better. And if we can find ways to let each other know that, through it all, we're in this together and together we'll get through it—it will help.

When my husband and I start to feel at odds, I will try to put myself in his shoes, and hope he can do the same for me.

No day is so bad it can't be fixed with a nap.
🦶 CARRIE SNOW

*W*hile we may fatigue easily during pregnancy, and fall asleep at the drop of a hat, the little baby factory inside our belly is on a twenty-four-hour nonstop shift. Perhaps that's why we suddenly find ourselves wide-awake in the middle of the night for no apparent reason. We don't have to go to the bathroom; we haven't been startled awake by a bad dream; and while we can feel our baby's movement, her kicks aren't strong enough to rouse us from a deep sleep.

Seasoned parents tell us that this type of wakefulness, known as "interrupted sleep," is common. Perhaps these wakeful intervals are preparing us for night feedings. Maybe they're giving us an opportunity to think about what we're getting into. Whatever the reason, we can use this time to catch up on our reading, reflect on the future, or simply count baby booties until we fall back to sleep.

My pregnant body is active twenty-four hours a day. When my sleep is interrupted, I will view it as a chance to engage in quiet, relaxing activities. Sleep will return soon enough.

Some questions don't have answers, which is a
terribly difficult lesson to learn.

♪ KATHARINE GRAHAM

For first-time mothers, discovering that there are a million questions for which there are no clear-cut answers can be nerve-racking. "How will I know when my water breaks?" or "How will I be able to tell the difference between my water breaking, vaginal discharge, and sweat if the amniotic fluid leaks out slowly instead of coming in one big gush?" Then there's the birth. "When should I call the midwife? Will my contractions really come five minutes apart? How can I be certain if I'm in labor or simply experiencing false labor?" The questions never end—and many answers only spawn more questions.

It is helpful to listen carefully to our doctor, and gather as much information as possible so when The Big Day comes we can trust that we know what to do.

I will prepare myself for the birth by getting as many answers to my questions as possible. Then I'll relax and trust myself and my own instincts.

Nothing in life is to be feared. It is only to be understood.

❧ MARIE CURIE

Gathering solid information about the birthing process can allay fears about the unknown. Like young children, we can ask "what if" questions to fill in the blanks. "What if I can't handle the pain? What are my options?" "What if my water breaks while I'm out shopping?" "What if my contractions come to a complete halt during labor?" Once we find answers to our questions, we will have a better understanding of the birthing process, and it won't seem as frightening.

The more information I receive from my physician, the less I will fear the upcoming birth.

I have two enormous dogs and they are both intimidated by my cat, Little Bits. Whenever she fearlessly rubs up against them, they freeze. I wonder what they'll act like when a baby comes crawling up to them!

👣 JESSE ACKERMAN

We often refer to our pets as our "children." We treat them like members of the family. But soon there will be a tiny human in the house and it will be interesting to see how they react. Like older siblings, they'll probably show signs of jealousy. They'll nudge us to remind us that they're being ignored. They'll carry their food dish out into the living room to announce the dinner hour. And they'll run from the room with tail tucked between legs whenever our infant wails.

We can help our pets adjust to the new member of the family by taking the time to introduce them properly, and by giving them the extra love they need during a difficult time for them, too.

I am not the only member of the household that will have to adjust to a new baby. I will need to introduce my pets to my child so they won't be afraid or feel left out.

Children are hopes.

♬ NOVALIS

*W*hen it comes to children, hope springs eternal. We envision the best for them. We wish them genuine happiness. We give them our best. By the same token, children keep our hope alive. When we feel beaten down by disappointment and things don't go as planned, our children's tender touch helps us to go on. If we are discouraged, their laughter lightens our load. They never give up on us; they never give up on life. That is what hope is all about.

My child will be like a bright candle that lights my way in the darkness.

Working together is a shared accomplishment.
❧ JODIE FOSTER

*M*any men today are experiencing the joys and challenges of raising children. No longer are the mundane tasks of picking up puzzle pieces, stacking the dishes in the cabinet, sterilizing the pacifiers, and wiping down the high chair tray considered "women's work." Men are sharing the load. Not only have they come to appreciate the amount of hard work involved in child rearing, but they have become part of the parenting team. And together, we are stronger.

**When my husband and I work as a team,
we lighten the load and reap the rewards
of family life.**

What did I think of pregnancy? I loved it. I could set my dinner plate on my stomach and eat while I watched TV in bed.

🐾 ANDIE MACDOWELL

*W*e usually hear about the negative aspects of pregnancy's final months: "I thought I was going to pop." "I couldn't find a comfortable position to sleep in." "I couldn't bend over, and I couldn't see my toes!" Nevertheless, consider the benefits. We can prop up our favorite book against our girth and read before going to sleep. And when it comes to eating in bed, no worries. We already come equipped with a tray.

My enlarged abdomen need not be a hindrance to life's little pleasures; it can be a help.

It is neither wise nor good to start a child with too much thought.

♫ COLETTE

*M*any a mother has spoken these very words after her first pregnancy, only to retract them at a later date: "After all that hard work, I'm not sure I could ever have another one." But nature has a wonderful way of giving us selective amnesia so we forget the less desirable aspects of pregnancy and birth. When we consider having a second or third child we will more than likely remember the positive things.

If I think too much about having another child, I might frighten myself out of it.

Become aware of how far you have already come. . . .
Realize that you have already accomplished much
more than you have imagined.

🌸 CAROLINE JOY ADAMS

*I*f you're like most women, you tend to focus
on those things you have yet to accomplish
instead of seeing how far you have already come.
But take a moment to think about all you have
done. Perhaps you completed your college degree.
Started your own business. Or perhaps you over-
came some financial obstacle or psychological diffi-
culty. Think what you are accomplishing now that
you are pregnant. You are creating a new being,
nourishing him within your womb, carrying him
until he is ready to be in the world. Celebrate your
accomplishments and remember that you have
what it takes to accomplish much more.

**I will take stock of my accomplishments and feel
good about how far I have come.**

It is a hard matter, my fellow citizens, to argue with the belly, since it has no ears.

PLUTARCH

*P*regnant women are notorious for craving sweets. We see a child licking a lollipop and we have to have one, too. We pass a neighborhood bakery en route to work and we feel compelled to stop and buy a pastry even if it means we'll be late. Anything resembling dessert catches our attention and we begin to salivate like Pavlov's dog! Our body seems to crave food devoid of nutritional value. And the cravings increase in direct proportion to our girth.

Just like an infant's, my cravings demand instant gratification.

With kicks like that my baby is destined to have an illustrious dance career ahead of him!

♫ JOI HAN

*I*sn't it amazing how active babies can be in utero? Their kicks can be strong and hard. Sometimes it seems as if they are dancing in our tummies with no concern for the fact that they just did the two-step on our bladders or a high kick into our ribs!

During the final months of pregnancy it seems that our child is destined to follow in the footsteps of Fred Astaire and Ginger Rogers. She's got happy feet that can't seem to wait to touch the earth.

Why does it seem that my baby kicks most vigorously as I'm about to fall asleep?

I would be curious to discover who it is to whom one writes in a diary. Possibly to some mysterious personification of one's own identity.

❧ BEATRICE WEBB

Keeping a pregnancy diary can be an illuminating way to chart a unique passage in our lives. Each day may be different from the next. We may be cognizant of a range of feelings: happiness because we will soon be a mother; anxiety because we fear we don't have a nurturing bone in our body; and awe as a new being forms within us. We may write from a more honest place within ourselves and discover a more daring and caring voice than the one we express to others.

I will record this special time on the pages of a journal so I may return to this conversation with myself in years to come.

*Nobody has ever measured, even poets, how much
the heart can hold.*

> ZELDA FITZGERALD

The experience of pregnancy can open the
most tender chambers of our hearts. We may
weep with joy as our baby rolls around inside of us.
We demonstrate our love by playing music, reading
poetry aloud, and gently cooing the sweetest of
sounds. Like teenagers, we experience the headi-
ness of falling in love.

With each passing month our love deepens. And
when our baby arrives, we will discover how
immeasurable our love truly is.

**My heart is so full of love, I feel I might burst
with joy!**

I'm lost! I've gone to look for myself. If I should return before I get back, please ask me to wait.

♪ A SIGN IN A CRAFT STORE, BEREA, KENTUCKY

*P*regnancy can turn our brains into mush. Some days we can't tell whether we're coming or going. We walk around in a daze, unable to focus. We try to concentrate on our daily tasks only to discover that we can't remember where we placed our list! When others become cross with us or impatient at our wanderings, all we have to do is remind them that we're pregnant and the combination of hormones and fatigue can make us forgetful. Hopefully, they will expect less from us until our memory returns.

Now is not the time to compete on game shows. I will maintain a sense of humor, knowing my condition may get worse before it gets better.

Fear had left me behind—it seemed the easiest thing in the world. All you had to do was give in. Yield and be taken.

❦ LYNNE SHARON SCHWARTZ

Isn't it wonderful to feel ready for whatever our baby's birth might bring? For many of us, this feeling occurs during the final months of pregnancy while we're attending a birthing class. For others, the fear leaves during a particular moment, possibly days before the birth, or in the midst of it.

When the fear is gone, we feel a strength: an inner preparedness that lets us know that everything is going to be okay.

If I release my fear, it will no longer have power over me.

I'm the worst person at keeping a secret, especially when it's a good secret I'm dyin' to tell.

🐾 ROSIE O'DONNELL

*J*t isn't easy to keep a secret, especially when the secret involves our pregnancy. In our excitement, we want to spread the news, ring the bells, and shout it from on high. But we wait until we are showing before we announce the news to family, friends, and coworkers "just in case."

While this is a sound strategy, not telling can sometimes be awkward. One expectant mother had to attend a wine tasting for work. Everyone noticed she wasn't tasting any of the quality wines offered, and some wondered if she had a drinking problem or if her religion prevented her from consuming liquor. Only later, when she revealed her pregnant condition, did the reason for her abstinence become clear.

Keeping my pregnancy a secret might produce some interesting speculation. Hopefully, it'll be of the entertaining variety.

Give a little love to a child and you get a great deal back.

♫JOHN RUSKIN

*I*t's not always easy to spend as much time as we would like with our children. Work, errands, even a new pregnancy, can interfere. Visits to the doctor, birthing class, and the need for more rest can make us less available.

While it is easy to feel guilty that we aren't as accessible to our children as we once were, the fact is, we have to take care of ourselves and follow our doctor's orders to ensure a healthy delivery. Talking to our children about their new baby sibling helps. We can also involve them in the pregnancy and make them feel special as the older brother and sister. Let them listen to the baby's heartbeat and feel his kicks, or take them on a shopping trip to buy a gift for the new baby. They could pick out crib sheets in *their* favorite color. This way, both our needs and theirs can be met simultaneously.

Being in tune with my children's needs is no guarantee that I can fulfill every one. But I can combine our needs in creative ways that are satisfying to all of us.

Before Erica was born I didn't have a clue about the different brands of baby products. Now I'm a pro.
❧ GINGER HINCHMAN-BIRKELAND

*B*ecoming a baby equipment consumer isn't easy. There's a lot to know! We can't tell the difference between brands. We don't understand the variance in prices. Heck, half the time, we're not even sure what we're looking at! It's like entering an alien world without a map. When we ask for assistance from the store clerks, they rattle off a bunch of information that only confuses us more. We'd probably be better off going to the experts: seasoned moms who know what's out there, what we need and what we don't, and where we can get the best deals.

It's hard to believe that soon I'll be one of those moms who can speak with authority on the quality of baby wipes, the pros and cons of pull-ups, the best strollers, and what to look for in cribs. But I will! And I'll be happy to help those who follow me.

Pregnancy often causes women to be forgetful. Concentrate on the funny side and laugh when "mother brain" causes you to put your keys in the refrigerator and garlic salt in your purse.

🦶 KAREN BRENDEL

*W*hile your body is working overtime on creating a new human being, occasionally precious mental resources may be diverted from their usual assignments. That's where the infamous "mother brain" of pregnancy comes from, and while it can be mildly embarrassing or annoying, it's also perfectly normal. Although it may be inconvenient to search for our keys, attempt to locate our purse for the third time today, or rack our brains over the latest bank deposit ("Did I or didn't I?"), thankfully, it is not fatal. We will recover our sharp memory and agile mind—if we can remember where we left it!

Forgetfulness can be a normal part of the pregnancy experience. I'll try to remember my sense of humor and see the humor in my gaffes.

The best-laid plans of mice and men go oft awry.
♫ ROBERT BURNS

*H*ard times can come even during pregnancy. Our future may not look as bright as we had hoped: our relationship might be foundering, our job situation may be uncertain, we may have concerns about our health or trouble finding a suitable yet affordable nanny. All our carefully laid plans appear to have been for naught. Everything seems to be going wrong and we don't know why.

In times like these, we need the support of friends and loved ones who can help us weather the storm until harmony—even if it's a different form of harmony than we had previously envisioned—is restored.

When things go wrong it isn't always my fault. My challenge is to make the best of whatever situation I am facing.

By and large, mothers and housewives are the only workers who do not have regular time off. They are the great vacationless class.
❧ ANNE MORROW LINDBERGH

*M*ost of us live in urban or suburban settings. Concrete and pavement are everywhere. Skyscrapers block the sun and commercial signs litter the highways. While the conveniences of city life are many, it is essential to escape urban sprawl every once in a while and return to paradise. It doesn't matter if we go to the Caribbean, the Canadian Rockies, or just to the nearest state park. Whichever destination we choose, it's good to be surrounded by pristine, untouched vistas.

While I am pregnant, I should consider a trip to paradise: an undeveloped place where I can take in the unobstructed beauty of nature and let it work its healing, restorative powers on me.

My mother had to be the bride at every wedding and the corpse at every funeral.

JOAN RIVERS

Sometimes it feels as though everyone wants to get in on the act. Our mother calls to tell us she's changed her work schedule so she can be present at our prenatal exams. Our father decides to give our car a tune-up since "we wouldn't want car trouble to ruin the big day." Then it's Aunt Sophie's turn—she insists on accompanying us on our first shopping trip since she was, after all, "the *only* one of the Edison girls to give birth to more than three children."

While well-meaning relatives want to be included in "the big nine months," we might need to remind them that a supporting role would be more helpful than competing for one of the leads.

I will welcome my family's contributions, doing my best to politely curb their intrusions.

The secret of life is not to get rid of the butterflies in
your stomach but to get them to fly in formation.
♫ ANONYMOUS

*T*ouring the hospital before birth is always a
good idea. Although it is natural to feel appre-
hensive at first, as though the butterflies in our
stomach are madly flapping their wings, it is good
to remember that the more familiar we become
with the sights, sounds, and smells of the delivery
room, the less daunting it will be. If we are brave
enough to look at the surgical instruments—forceps,
syringes, and oxygen tanks—just seeing them up
close can reduce our anxiety.

Childbirth preparation classes are also very helpful in getting both ourselves and our coach prepared for the labor ahead. The more knowledge we
have, the better prepared we'll be for a good and
safe birth. Who knows? We might even enjoy it!

Familiarizing myself with those things that are
causing my fear is the best way to overcome it.

*My advice to you is not to inquire why or whither,
but just enjoy your ice cream while it's on your plate.*
❧ THORNTON NIVEN WILDER

*N*ot a bad philosophy, is it? When we find
ourselves going 'round and 'round over the
same question without reaching an answer, it's time
to leave it alone. Sometimes when we "switch
tracks" and are thinking about something
completely different, we will unexpectedly arrive
at an answer. In the meantime, why don't we just
enjoy what's on our plate, trusting that the question
will return with greater clarity when our minds have
had a break.

**Questions, like babies, need time to gestate
before they can be born. Otherwise, the outcome
will be "premature."**

The first day of spring was once the time for taking the young virgins into the fields, there in dalliance to set an example in fertility for Nature to follow. Now we just set the clock an hour ahead and change the oil in the crankcase.

👣 E.B. WHITE

*W*e all get into a rut sometimes. Yet when we are expecting, our energy can diminish and we can become overly focused on accomplishing everything before the baby arrives. We simply aren't in the right frame of mind to think about spicing things up. Isn't it wonderful, then, when our husband takes it upon himself to whisk us away to a nearby resort? Perhaps we can go hiking for a couple of days, or soak in mineral waters at a spa and order all our meals from room service. If that doesn't suit our fancy, perhaps we can go out dancing at the local club, visit a special museum exhibit, or take in a play.

Adding spice to life makes me feel better all the way around.

When she stopped conforming to the conventional picture of femininity, she finally began enjoying being a woman.

♫ BETTY FRIEDAN

S ocietal definitions of pregnancy can have a direct impact on an expectant mother's psyche. For example, parental leave is still defined as "disability leave," as though pregnancy is an abnormal medical condition. Our pregnancy may bring into question the conventional and outdated notion that pregnancy (due to its sexual nature) should be concealed. And if we wear a bikini in public like pregnant women in Europe do, allowing our belly to be visible to the world, we may be viewed as indecent or scandalous.

I feel radiant and full. I will let myself shine forth like the round, full moon.

Before your wife begins to show, you may have to break the news to an older sibling that a charming stranger will be moving into your house who's going to get maximum attention from all living creatures for the next several years, destroy the family's sleep, throw food at random objects, and drool onto all nearby shoulders.

❦ JAMES DOUGLAS BARRON

I'll never forget the words of an instructor in a mother and baby class I took when Alexander was just six months old. She laid it on the line: "For those of you who are already contemplating your second child, and expecting your oldest to be thrilled with a new baby brother or sister, let me put it this way. If your husband came home one day and enthusiastically announced to you that he was going to bring a new wife into the house, and that 'you'd just love her,' what do you think your reaction would be?" Her words gave us pause. "I never thought of it that way," one mother said. "Well, you might want to start," the instructor replied.

It's wise to remember that my older children may not be as thrilled about a new baby as I am—at least initially. In time, the bonds will form.

Most beds sleep up to six cats. Ten without the owner.
🐾 ENGLISH PROVERB

C ats love to sleep with pregnant women. And why wouldn't they? We radiate incredible heat to warm the covers in winter. Our tummy provides a perch on which they can drape themselves and take a nap. Their purring feels so good against our taut muscles that we spend long stretches of time scratching under its chin. The only downside (for the cat): to have its snooze rudely interrupted by our frequent need to get up to pee.

Together, my cat and I will make the best use of my bed.

When I dare to be powerful, to use my strength in the service of my vision, then it becomes less and less important whether or not I am afraid.

♫ AUDRE LORDE

*I*s there ever a perfect time to become a mother? Probably not. Millionaires lose their fortunes overnight, job security can vanish with a company merger, and promotions don't materialize as expected. Yet isn't it nice to know that regardless of external disappointments and unanticipated changes, we have held fast to our conviction? We have always dreamt of becoming a mother. And now we stand at the threshold of realizing our vision. What a tremendous achievement!

My fear will shrink next to the strength of my convictions. I am going to be a mother!

Three reasons to exercise during pregnancy:
1. *To keep your ass from sagging*
2. *To get into shape so labor will only seem like one more marathon you're capable of finishing*
3. *Pregnant women look cute in sportswear*

🌺 LORRIE GOLDBERG

*E*xpectant mothers sometimes become too serious about exercise. We think of it as a cure-all for any physical shortcomings, even those that existed *before* we got pregnant. We become unrealistic, thinking that with enough regimented and vigorous exercise we can have the ultimate body we've always wanted and avoid the natural consequences of pregnancy.

While safe and moderate exercise during pregnancy is a good thing, worrying about how to get our pre-pregnancy shape back is not. Before we become obsessed and buy a closetful of maternity sportswear, we'd better take a sanity check and realize that drooping breasts, an enlarged abdomen, and a sagging behind are better tackled *after* the baby is born.

Sometimes I need a better sense of humor, not more exercise, to keep my self in shape.

There are two lasting bequests we can hope to give our children. One is roots; the other, wings.

HODDING CARTER

otherhood pulls us in opposite directions. We must be protective and loving so our child may know his roots are deep and strong. Yet at the same time, we must encourage his steps toward autonomy. We must stick to our word so our child has faith in us, while we encourage him to trust himself. We must also be generous with our guidance and discipline so that one day our child will no longer need them and will soar out into the world with confidence.

Starting with my pregnancy, I will build a strong foundation for my child.

One hour with a child is like a ten-mile run.
JOAN BENOIT SAMUELSON, MARATHON RUNNER

eeping a child bathed, fed, and amused can be more challenging than running a marathon. We are in constant motion preparing bottles, changing diapers, winding toys, and fetching teething rings. It's hard work. But just like a runner, we'll put one foot in front of the other and pray for pit stops.

My child will take as much energy as a ten-mile run. I'd better build my stamina now.

Every child is born a genius.

❧ R. BUCKMINSTER FULLER

*B*uckminster Fuller had incredible faith in humankind. He recognized the innate intelligence in children and their potential for achieving great things. Forever the optimist, Fuller believed there was no limit to the human intellect. In his eyes no child was ever dull or dim-witted. Adults need only provide encouragement and every child would shine.

My child will have a special kind of genius all her own. I will help her carry it into the world.

Mighty is the force of motherhood!
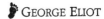 GEORGE ELIOT

*R*ight about now we're sensing the indescribable force of motherhood. Before our baby has exited the womb we feel like Dorothy in *The Wizard of Oz* saying to her dog, Toto, "I don't think we're in Kansas anymore." It's as though we've landed in a strange land that is both inviting and frightening. Our psyche can't completely comprehend the changes we are experiencing. Yet, undoubtedly, we have entered new territory. And, just like Dorothy's, our journey will be full of adventures and surprises.

Motherhood is an impressive force that will bend and shape me: a new woman is being born.

There is nothing as easy as denouncing. It don't take much to see that something is wrong, but it takes some eyesight to see what will put it right again.

♫ WILL ROGERS

If we find ourselves constantly complaining about our husband's lack of involvement with the pregnancy, we'd better do something about it right away. He may not know how to join in. He might feel inadequate or out of place. Perhaps he thinks of pregnancy as "a woman's thing" and assumes he should stay out of it.

Instead of letting resentment build up, why don't we tell him how we feel? Why don't we give him the opportunity to take part in the pregnancy, even if it is only to drive to the store in the middle of the night to get us ice cream? If, on the other hand, he seems resistant to participating, we would do well to talk about the problem now, before the baby arrives and we are too tired and worn out to do so.

Rather than denouncing my husband for his lack of sensitivity and involvement, I can go about trying to set things right.

I feel like a stranger in a strange land.

❧ ROBERT A. HEINLEIN

*H*ave you ever walked into an exclusive men's club and felt like a total alien? That's probably how our husbands feel when they first enter a gynecological examining room. The plastic pelvic model looks like a relic from high school science. Calendars with advertisements for birth control pills paper the walls. And when it comes to picking a seat, they have to choose between a short stool on rollers or the exam table—both unfitting options.

To help our husband feel more comfortable in the female medical scene, we can describe the procedure ahead of time, make sure he has one-on-one time with our OB-GYN to discuss his concerns and ask questions. And, most important, we can assure him that pregnancy is not the exclusive domain of women. There's a place for him.

I will be sensitive to the ways that husbands are made to feel like outsiders and include and involve my husband in our pregnancy.

You can't look at a sleeping cat and feel tense.
🐾 JANE PAULEY

*I*sn't it wonderful to lie in bed with a cat purring on our pregnant tummy? Like a heating pad with fur, he relaxes our tired muscles and smooths out the tired knots. He makes our eyelids droop, and we wonder, "When he purrs, can my baby hear him? Does my little one feel the gentle kneading of my cat's mini massage? Is it relaxing to him, too?" Hopefully, the answer is yes.

I will follow my cat's example, do a leisurely cat stretch, then curl up and go limp.

*An intense feeling carries with it its own universe,
magnificent or wretched as the case may be.*

♫ ALBERT CAMUS

*P*regnancy is a world unto itself. We are
suddenly thrust into a sea of emotions and
bodily changes that, until now, may have been
foreign to us. Sometimes these all-consuming feelings make us feel isolated because others are too
engrossed in the busyness of their own lives to
share them. They may not relate to our comments
about the tenderness of our breasts or the occa-
sional cramping of our uterus.

At times, pregnancy can feel lonely as though no
one else understands what we're going through. At
other times, we can cocoon ourselves within the
experience, gladly removing ourselves from the
more mundane concerns of the external world.

**Pregnancy is my universe right now. I will soak
in its experiences.**

The logic of the heart is absurd.

🌱 JULIE DE LESPINASSE

*A*s expectant mothers, we sometimes go a bit overboard making sure our baby has the best of everything. We shop at twenty stores for the most solid crib. We research strollers for ratings on safety and convenience. We buy multiple outfits, forgetting that they will last only a week or two. And we fill the nursery dresser drawers with the most adorable sleepers, patterned with cuddly bunnies and Holstein cow designs. The truth is, we're already so pathetically in love with this tiny being that we've lost all practicality and are led only by the generosity of our heart.

The logic of the heart may be as absurd as it is wonderful.

Be willing to know what you know.

> CHARLOTTE DAVIS KASL

From the moment of conception, I knew my child was going to be a boy. I just *knew* it. Yet, throughout my pregnancy, everyone would refer to the being inside of me as "she." In the final months of pregnancy I was weary of correcting friends and complete strangers, so I allowed others to refer to my child with whatever pronoun they wished.

Then, during my emergency C-section, seconds before the incision was made, I heard the doctor say to me, "She'll be coming out soon." Unable to help myself, I made one last correction. "It's a boy, not a girl!" I told her emphatically. And when the baby popped out, wasn't everyone surprised. She had a penis!

I will trust my instincts and not allow others to talk me out of them.

*I never close my door behind me without the aware-
ness that I am carrying out an act of mercy toward
myself.*

♫ PETER HOEG

s pregnant women we need to give ourselves moments of solitude and quiet. Pregnancy takes a lot out of us, and motherhood will
demand even more. Why not do ourselves a favor
and take time for ourselves, closing the door to
outside noise and distractions. Otherwise, our body
and spirit will be depleted; instead of enjoying pregnancy, it will feel like a burden.

The next time the busy hum of the outer world
becomes overwhelming, why not shut the hustle
and bustle out and go inside for a while?

**I will create a sanctuary for myself today. It is an
act of mercy.**

Some folks are natural born kickers. They can always find a way to turn disaster into butter.

         🌸 KATHERINE PATERSON

*I*sn't it great to have positive support from those around us? Whenever we worry that we aren't eating exactly right, our friends help us to take a more realistic approach. Whenever we get down in the dumps believing that we'll be the worst mother on earth, they hold our hands and soothe our tears until we gain a better perspective. They always seem to look on the bright side and console us with their optimism. What would we do without them?

Whenever everything looks gloomy, I'll look to those friends who can help me see the positive side.

Ideas won't keep: something must be done about them.

ALFRED NORTH WHITEHEAD

*B*ecoming a mother can awaken passions in us we have ignored until now. We may feel inspired to open a bakery shop we had always hoped for, or we might feel compelled to return to school to complete our master's degree. Perhaps it's time to quit an unfulfilling job or change apartments or redecorate our house or paint a portrait or . . .

The fact is, pregnancy can open other creative channels in us that have been dormant. Although it is likely that others may caution against our taking on new things, since we will soon have our hands full, for some of us, pregnancy may be the spur to a creative change we need.

Pregnancy may be just the catalyst I need to forge ahead with passionate endeavors.

When the student is ready, the teacher will appear.

♫ ZEN PROVERB

The life passage we are now entering will test us, teach us, and give us knowledge—sometimes through joy, sometimes through fire. Rather than reinvent the wheel, why not learn from those who have traversed this path before? We might just be surprised at how much our own mother (or a friend's mother) knows.

Knowing when the teacher appears is half the challenge. Being open to the lessons offered is the other half.

Sages, mentors, and teachers will appear on the road of pregnancy. Hopefully, I will be a good student.

*Never before have I had to be so aware of my body
and my relationship to it.*

🦶 LYNN HARRISON

*I*f we strain a muscle during pregnancy, we
feel it. If we stand on our feet too long, we
notice the discomfort. Pregnancy makes us acutely
aware of the rigors we put our bodies through day
in and day out. For a time, we may have to "baby"
an old injury that is acting up. Or we may need to
have our feet rubbed periodically to reduce the
swelling. The fact is, we are not machines. Pregnancy puts a tremendous strain on our system, and
if we attempt to ignore our body's messages, we
will wear it out and run it down.

**The aches and pains are my body's way of telling
me it needs attention. I will heed them.**

*It is the belief in a power larger than myself and
other than myself . . . which allows me to venture into
the unknown and even the unknowable.*

♪ MAYA ANGELOU

*R*egardless of our religious beliefs, pregnancy
brings us face-to-face with the power of the
unknown. Although we can describe conception
and the splitting of the cells in scientific terms, the
miracle of pregnancy is a deeply felt reality. Being
pregnant means participating in the mystery of this
miracle. Becoming a mother takes tremendous faith.
We don't know what the future will bring. We don't
know how our child will turn out. All we can do is
trust our partner, God, and ourselves as we forge a
path into the unknown.

**As a mother once said: "Becoming a mother is
the ultimate act of faith. There are so many
unknowns, and there are no guarantees. Only
hope."**

*Everybody gets so much information all day long
that they lose their common sense.*

🌸 GERTRUDE STEIN

*A*n exasperated mother once remarked:
"Reading all these books on pregnancy, I've
learned more than I ever cared to think about." Many
expectant mothers share those sentiments. And yet we
worry that we're not preparing properly if we don't
read every book on the pediatrician's library shelf. We
wonder which advice applies and how much we need
to know. We discover interesting facts we'd never
heard of, and wonder what else we might be missing
in our database.

To make things easier, it helps to have a recommended reading list from our physician or midwife.
We can ask mothers we admire to recommend books
they found most useful. Or if we are involved in a
childbirth class, we might ask our instructor for perti-
nent reading material. Limiting our reading to a few
good books and articles can give us enough of the
information we need without the overload.

**Pregnancy can be a research project in and of
itself. I will be selective about the material I
choose to read.**

Progress does not come without its costs.
> E. F. SCHUMACHER

Not only do we expectant mothers have to watch our diets, nowadays we also have to be careful of the chemicals and additives in foods. Rather than obsessing over the foods we prepare, why not keep it simple and safe? Choose fresh foods over processed ones and, whenever possible, eat organic produce and chemical-free meat and dairy products. That way, we can ensure sound health for our baby, and ourselves.

Whenever I can, I will eat fresh, not processed, foods, and when in doubt, I'll check the ingredients out.

Dictators are rulers who always look good until the last ten minutes.

♫ JAN MASARYK

How do you feel about your current obstetrician? Does he ask for your input? Does she answer your questions to your satisfaction? Does he dictate how the birth will be or is he interested in assisting you with the type of birth you would like to have?

If you have any concerns about your physician, now is the time to address them. Don't be afraid to "change horses" even if the medical community advises against it. The fact is, if you feel safe and secure with your doctor, you will be more relaxed during the birthing process. And if things don't go as planned, you'll feel more secure in the hands of someone you trust.

It is important to have a physician I feel comfortable with for the birth of my baby. I will take the time to find a doctor who respects my wishes.

*An unhurried woman is willing to include some
emptiness in her day. That way, when you ask if she's
got time for you, she almost always does.*

        ✿ VICTORIA MORAN

*R*emember when you were a child and there
was one house in the neighborhood where
everyone liked to congregate? Why? Because an
unhurried woman lived inside. She had time to
listen to the events of your life: the latest crush on a
curly-haired boy; the gossip circulating around the
school yard; inner musings about your plans for the
future. And when dinner came out of the oven, she
simply set an extra place at the table and told you to
pull up a seat.

    Although our lives seem more complicated than
that of the unhurried woman from our past, we
would do well to remember her example. Soon we
will have a little one whose needs will demand that
we slow down and make unhurried time for her.

**If I include some unhurried time in my day, my
child will feel that I have time for her and
whatever comes up.**

*O human race, born to fly upward, wherefore at a
little wind dost thou so fall?*

> DANTE ALIGHIERI

*P*eriodically, pregnancy can make us feel
more fragile than at other times in our lives,
and at a certain point we may notice that we are not
handling hardships well. Just a few months earlier
we thought we had the tiger by the tail; now we are
filled with doubt and confusion. We feel sensitive to
criticism, overwhelmed by pushy people, and our
tolerance for jerks is virtually nonexistent.

It is important to remember that these feelings are
normal. While they might not last long, we might
want our partner to protect us during these times.
He can run interference during family disputes,
derail aggressive salesmen on our behalf, and deal
with unkind flight attendants while in the air. And
when we need some extra reassurance, we can ask
to be held in the circle of his arms.

**Fragile states may come and go. I will make a
point of surrounding myself with those people
who are gentle with me right now.**

Housework can kill you, so why take the chance?
♫ ANONYMOUS

The more children we bring into the world, the more challenging it becomes to keep a clean house. Especially after the second or third child, we may not try as hard to stay on top of the mess because we know that within half an hour everything is going to look the way it did before.

It's more important than anything else to get plenty of rest when you're pregnant. Learn to ignore the voice of guilt, the imaginary whispers of others, and anything else that gets in the way of your nourishing your baby. If you can get help with the housework, do. If you can't, let it go.

In my pregnant state my energy may be limited. I will choose my priorities carefully. Housework may not be at the top of my list right now, and that's okay.

Endurance

The most despairing songs are the loveliest of all; I know immortal ones composed only of tears.

🌸 ALFRED DE MUSSET

Getting pregnant is not always easy. We may have to endure surgery, a battery of tests, only to be plagued by nagging questions such as "What's wrong with me?" before we finally conceive. Yet when we do become pregnant we do not take it for granted. It feels so incredibly precious and hard-earned that we savor every moment. We thank God for the miracle we tried so hard to create. The pain was worth it.

Isn't it nice to discover that when I ask myself if I had to do it all over again, I can answer with confidence, "Yes!"

No snowflake in an avalanche ever feels responsible.
STANISLAW JERZY LEC

*E*ver notice how the same philosophy applies to children? Whenever there's a catastrophe —pots and pans come tumbling out of the kitchen cabinet—they act as though it was an unexplainable occurrence. Pregnancy is a good time to encourage older children to take more responsibility for accidents and messes. Soon enough they will have to understand that Mommy will be busy with the newest member of the family and she cannot always stop what she's doing to rush to their aid. Not only will they learn a little self-sufficiency, but they'll be able to pitch in and contribute to the household.

There's no time like the present to teach my brood to be a little more self-sufficient. We will all benefit in the end.

If a man cares not for his roots, then how can he care for his branches?

♫ DOYLE M. DAVIS

No matter what our heritage, it is important to share our ethnic and cultural background with our children. It gives them a sense of pride, a shared identity, and a history in which to anchor themselves. If, in the past, our roots were not particularly important to us, we may experience a renewed sense of continuity with our ancestors when our own children are born. Being on the threshold of parenthood can make us more aware of the rich traditions that have been passed on through the centuries. We are continuing the lineage and, no doubt, our children will be richer for knowing the kin they came from.

Pregnancy can renew my sense of belonging to a unique family heritage. I will take time to get to know my relatives so I might pass on their legacies.

There are people who have money and people who are rich.

❀ COCO CHANEL

*P*regnancy reminds us that money isn't the only way to create wealth. The gift of children is precious, indeed. And although they come with expenses, they are worth it. In fact, having a child often helps us to realign our financial priorities and to measure the value of money differently. We learn to put people before things and we are repaid in love and kindness.

My money does not make me rich. My family does.

In this period she learns the discipline of sacrifice: her body, her time, her nutrients, her psyche, her knowledge, her skills, her social life, her economic capabilities, her relationships, and her spiritual knowledge and values are all called into the service of her children. This passage, ambivalent at best, pushes her to reach beyond whatever limits she thought she labored within, making her stronger. . . .

PAULA GUNN ALLEN

Motherhood is a powerful transformation. That is why we are given nine months to prepare. Every aspect of who we are is called into service for our child, and we quickly discover our weaknesses, our lack of knowledge, and just how capable we are, especially in the face of adversity. Unfortunately, children don't come with operating instructions. Sometimes we're learning from scratch and other times we can build on the skills we have. But we're always exploring new talents that will enable us to be more effective mothers.

Motherhood will call on all my strengths and talents. I will heed the call.

It is not enough to have a good mind. The main thing is to use it well.

♪ RENÉ DESCARTES

*P*regnancy can put our minds to the test. We have to make informed choices throughout our entire pregnancy. Even simple decisions like taking a pain reliever for a headache cannot be taken for granted. We must be aware of any potentially harmful effects aspirin, Tylenol, or Advil might have on our growing baby. When our doctor or midwife asks us what type of medication we would choose if we need assistance during labor, we research it. . . . Before we know it, we are experts on pharmaceuticals, biology, physiology, and obstetrics.

I have a good mind. I will use it to make informed decisions for my baby and myself.

Death, taxes, and childbirth? There's never a convenient time for any of them.

🌸 MARGARET MITCHELL

hildbirth might be convenient for our baby, but rarely is it convenient for us. We might have a board meeting scheduled that has to be canceled at the last minute, a business trip overseas, a family holiday function, or a plan to paint the house. It doesn't matter what is on our schedule. When our baby is ready, she's ready—and she doesn't care what we've got planned!

My child may not come at a convenient time for me, but it is right for her and I must respect her timing.

When I found I had crossed that line, I looked at my hands to see if I was the same person. There was such a glory over everything.

🦶 HARRIET TUBMAN

*H*arriet Tubman was a courageous woman who escaped the bonds of slavery to cross over into the free land. She had tremendous determination and perseverance. Although we may not think of ourselves as heroes, how many of us found the journey to motherhood to be a rough road? Yet we persisted until we finally crossed the line. Did we not feel there was "glory over everything" even if we could barely comprehend our success? Whether we endured the trials of infertility, the disappointment of miscarriage, or the stress of a prolonged adoption, we have all acted with courage and a resolute character.

The process of becoming a mother was more difficult than I could have imagined. Yet there was such glory when it happened.

Familiar acts are beautiful through love.

♪ PERCY BYSSHE SHELLEY

*I*sn't it wonderful when our beloved notices when we're flagging and achy and makes us a cup of tea? Or the laundry is washed and folded while we are getting dinner?

When we are pregnant, these thoughtful, simple acts can make all the difference. Instead of constantly keeping track of the household chores, we can concentrate on preparing for our new arrival. We can take time to work out at the gym, go for a walk in the hills, or simply close our eyes and listen to Mozart because, through these familiar, loving acts, we are given more time for other activities.

Familiar acts give me the gift of time. I feel cherished, loved, and appreciated.

Put not your trust in money, but your money in trust.
❧ OLIVER WENDELL HOLMES

Nowadays it seems we must begin saving for college before our child is born! The cost of raising a child is growing exponentially, and if she wants to attend a good university, the expenses can outdistance our bank accounts. Certainly, when we are pregnant, sending "our baby" to college seems incredibly far off in the future. But think again. As our parents always said, "They grow up so fast." College will be a reality sooner than we could have imagined.

Today, I will begin saving money for my child's education, even if it is only in small amounts.

Fear of Becoming a Father

With all the pain of it, I long for the wonderful thing to happen, for a tiny human creature to spring from between my limbs bravely out into the world.

👣 YANG PING

We may be thrilled about the prospect of becoming a mother, but our husband may not initially share that enthusiasm. Rather than focusing on the rewarding aspects of parenthood, he may be thinking about all the freedom he is going to lose and the responsibilities he'll have to assume. Whenever we attempt to verbalize our own excitement, hoping he'll join in, he looks like "a deer in headlights," paralyzed with fear.

While it may take him time to "come around," we need not take his feelings personally. Like us, he is going through enormous changes at the prospect of becoming a parent. And since he cannot know the experience of having a baby growing inside of him, it may take him longer to have the fear replaced by excitement. Until then, it is best if we can be compassionate and understanding.

I must be patient with my husband while he sorts through his fears and trepidation.

Curiosity is one of the permanent and certain characteristics of a vigorous mind.

♫ SAMUEL JOHNSON

*C*hances are, the pile of books on the nightstand are all about pregnancy. Since we're so steeped in the subject, why not explore the way childbirth and pregnancy are experienced in other cultures—whether in Africa, Bali, or South America. For example, in Africa, a Chagga father is taken aside and taught by the community of elders how to treat his pregnant wife. He is responsible for creating a calm atmosphere and protecting his wife from anger or violence. In Nigeria, expectant mothers are discouraged from quarreling or engaging in vicious gossip. Ibo women even cover their navel so the baby won't be exposed to harmful words and disturbing sights. In Japan, Tai-kyo, or embryonic education, stresses the need for harmony, asserting that the voices, thoughts, and feelings of the mother and father greatly influence the fetus.

I will explore birthing traditions from different cultures to see what I might want to incorporate into my own pregnancy.

The desire to take medicine is perhaps the greatest feature which distinguishes man from animals.

❧ SIR WILLIAM OSLER

*L*et's be honest, some of us have no tolerance for pain. We don't want to feel "the ring of fire" as our baby's head crowns. We don't want to breathe through every contraction. We aren't especially brave, and don't feel the need to be heroic during the final stages of delivery. We have nothing to prove. We want medication at the first hint of pain, and if our doctor doesn't give it to us we just might be forced to hurt him!

If I have a low tolerance for pain, I'd better let my doctor know in advance.

A people without history is like the wind on buffalo grass

👣 SIOUX ADAGE

Not so long ago, adoptions were conducted completely in private. The birth parents' names were never revealed and a child could not obtain information about them. For those of us who were adopted, the birth of our own child can present some unique challenges. Even if we wanted to, we cannot tell our child that he or she looks like Ompah or Aunt Bessie simply because we do not know. We are mothers without a biological or ancestral history. We must fill in our own life stories with the rich experiences we've had and, with our child, patch together our history as a family.

As an adopted child, I have to write my own history. With a child on the way, a new chapter is beginning.

I'm so fertile, I can get pregnant simply by folding my husband's underwear!

♫ JENNIFER BEST

ome of us get pregnant at the drop of a hat. It's as though our bodies defy the laws of physics, and no matter what we do, we end up pregnant. It doesn't matter if we use the pill, a diaphragm, condoms, or a combination thereof, if we miss one day of our period, we begin knitting booties!

I have to come to terms with the fact that I'm a "fertile turtle." Maybe now is the time to decide how many children we want so that when the magic number is reached my husband and I can consider a more permanent birth control method.

I thought I was finished having babies. My kids were in high school, my career was thriving, and my life felt complete. Then, poof, Max arrived.

🌸 MADELINE GERNSEY

*L*ife is full of surprises. And one of the biggest surprises is taking a home pregnancy test only to find that the result is positive! We didn't see it coming. We didn't plan it, and now here we are, in the midst of pregnancy again.

At first, we might experience mixed emotions: shock, happiness, doubt, fear, elation, excitement, and worry. Then as we reframe our thoughts in the next few weeks and call a family meeting, we find we can make room for this baby, and we welcome him into our hearts.

Life is full of surprises. I just happen to be carrying one of them inside of me!

*All the world is queer save me and thee; and
sometimes I think even thee is a little queer.*

QUAKER SPEAKING TO HIS WIFE

None of us likes to think of ourselves as
odd. But the fact is, we all possess eccen-
tricities. While we might conceal them from the
general public, our family members know us all too
well. Sure, they love us, but they know we can be
downright weird. Isn't it wonderful to know that we
will soon be adding another little person to our cast
of characters?

**My child might not know it yet, but he has been
recruited into a three-ring circus that I call home.**

If this is the best of all possible worlds, what are the others like?

♫ VOLTAIRE

*J*s something amiss? Does the life you have created feel foreign to you? Does it no longer feel like home? When we find ourselves feeling negative about our environment and the life we've built, it's time to make a change. Perhaps we're not the same person we once were. Maybe we've moved into a new phase of our life and we want our inner changes to be reflected in our outer environment.

Pregnancy can accentuate the need for a new world; a better world with a better fit for who we are *now*.

Whether I make a drastic change or a simple one, I can alter my world in ways that are reflective of who I am, who I have become, and who I want to be with my child.

It takes courage to be an unhurried woman. It means giving up accolades like, "I don't know how she does it all."

❧ VICTORIA MORAN

Sound familiar? Many of us in our childbearing years have thrived on a fast-paced, hectic schedule in pursuit of our professional goals. We always carry a cell phone, schedule our appointments dangerously close together, and multitask like there's no tomorrow.

Now that we're pregnant, we may want to rethink our priorities. If we continue at this pace when our child asks us for a hug, wants us to look at a picture he's painted, or needs help assembling a model airplane, our attention will be elsewhere. Perhaps we can learn to downshift when we come home from the office, and go into receptive mode.

My professional pace is great at the office, but my patient touch is what's needed at home.

The month of May was come, when every lusty heart beginneth to blossom, and to bring forth fruit. . . .
🐾 SIR THOMAS MALORY

*W*hen our maternal instincts kick in, they kick in. We want to get pregnant—NOW! But with two preschoolers in the house, it isn't always easy to conceive. They may start off sleeping in their own beds, but too often they end up sleeping in ours. And when we carry them back to their own room, they awaken and can't fall back to sleep. Privacy is as rare as the Hope diamond, and as precious. Who would have ever thought that our children would be the biggest obstacles to having more children?

I am ready to be pollinated so I can blossom and bring forth fruit. If my husband and I could only get a little time to ourselves . . .

Are we having fun yet?

♪ BILL GRIFFITH

*B*irthing classes can be hard work. There is so much to learn in such a short time that it feels like being back in college cramming for exams. We try to remember phase one and two, but we keep getting it mixed up with phase three. Or is there a phase three? And when do we take the short, panting breaths? And when the slow, deep ones?

The best we can do is take notes, review them with our partner, and hope we remember the important stuff when the time comes.

How can learning to deliver a baby be so funny and frustrating at the same time? I will continue to attend birthing class in hopes of finding out.

Every person takes the limits of his own field of vision for the limits of the world.
🌸 ARTHUR SCHOPENHAUER

None of us likes to think of ourselves as living in a box, but we do. We become comfortable in our belief system and there we stay until something breaks us out of it or we have a revelation that alters our perception.

Children stretch us. If we are receptive, they can change our views and help us to expand the limits of our world.

I will be open to seeing new vistas through my children's eyes, knowing that each child I bring into the world will open new worlds to me.

As a child I was always running late; why, I was even late for my own birthday.

RICH LITTLE

No one ever explained punctuality to kids. They simply never arrive on time. It doesn't matter whether our physician or midwife makes calculations based on our last period or the day of conception. A guess is still a guess, even if it is an educated one.

I won't count on my baby arriving on time. He'll choose his own birthday.

*Remember that the most beautiful things in the world
are the most useless: peacocks and lilies, for example.*
♪JOHN RUSKIN

e live in a pragmatic society that attributes
a low value to anything that is not useful.
Beautiful things are often viewed as frivolous orna-
mentation; but the truth is, beautiful things inspire
us, they feed our souls. When our body is weary, a
colorful picture can refresh us or a lavender-flax
pillow can help us relax. Simply placing a flower in
our hair can brighten our day. What could be worth
more than that?

**I will surround myself with beautiful things to
enhance this special time of my life.**

If life had a second edition, how would I correct the proofs?

🌸 JOHN CLARE

I always feel a little sorry for first children because they are given the task of breaking in their parents. And, as we know with first efforts, there are bound to be mistakes. Fortunately, we can learn from our mistakes. Not only can we become better parents for our second and third child, but we can modify our parenting style in such a way that all our children benefit. As one mother expressed it: "I want to be a second-time mother, the first time around."

I can fine-tune my mothering style any time.

I never forget a face, but in your case, I'll make an exception.

🦶 GROUCHO MARX

Have you ever had to have a blood test or urine analysis and been treated by the nurse-from-hell? You know the one. She makes snide comments about the weight you've gained. She isn't particularly gentle with the needle. And when you ask her what to do with your urine sample, she looks at you as if she expects you to drink it! Probably the best thing to do is ignore her rudeness or, perhaps, give her a dose of her own medicine.

Luckily, most of the medical professionals I deal with are kind and considerate. I won't let one spoiled apple ruin the whole bunch or my day.

I believe in the discipline of silence and could talk about it for hours.

♫ GEORGE BERNARD SHAW

*I*n order to still our mind and fully relax our body, we need silence. We need a space and time simply to be—without the interference of a television blaring or car engines and horns jarring our brains. But it isn't always easy to keep the silence once we've attained it. Instead of emptying our minds, we think about all the friends whose phone calls we have to return. We remember the name of the new restaurant we wanted to tell our mother about, and before we know it, our mouths are moving again.

Silence takes discipline. I will resist the temptation to engage in distractions that pull me away from my peace.

Dwelling on the negative simply contributes to its power.

🌸 SHIRLEY MACLAINE

We all go through times when we focus only on those things that are going wrong. "My maternity clothes make me look like a bloated fish," we moan. Or, "My face is breaking out. I look worse than I did when I was a teenager!" We even gripe about events that haven't yet transpired: "I doubt I'll ever be able to get to the gym once the baby arrives."

When we focus solely on the negative, the world looks bleak. We forget about all the things that are going right. What if we took a moment to write down a list of all the things we're grateful for? Surely, they would counterbalance the disappointments and aggravations, helping us to gain a more realistic—and happier—perspective.

When I open my eyes to the positive aspects of pregnancy, I break the negative cycle.

As a matter of biology, if something bites you it is probably female.

SCOTT M. KRUSE

*P*regnant women are known for sinking their teeth into things. When hit by a sudden craving, we bite into a piece of chocolate, but it doesn't satisfy our impulse. We chomp on a carrot, but it tastes too healthy. Like a teething puppy, we need some relief—and so we pounce on our husband and nibble on his neck.

I can't help it. Sometimes a love bite is the only way to quell my oral urges!

Amoebas at the start were not complex;
They tore them apart and started sex.

♫ ARTHUR GUITERMAN

Sex during pregnancy can be fraught with mixed feelings. We worry that intercourse might harm the baby. Our rampant hormones make us feel amorous one day and standoffish the next. Our spouse might have conflicting feelings about being passionate with us now that he has begun to perceive us as a mother. Sometimes we end up feeling hurt and rejected, while he suffers from feelings he doesn't understand and struggles to overcome the obstacles that prevent him from expressing his love.

As a couple, we should talk about these difficult feelings. Otherwise they get buried and grow larger until they overshadow the satisfying union we once shared. Even if we don't end up having sex, at least we can feel close at a time when it's so essential.

Sex during pregnancy need not be complicated if my partner and I are willing to share our feelings openly and honestly—even the ones we feel might hurt.

The most beautiful thing we can experience is the mysterious.

🌸 ALBERT EINSTEIN

*U*ntil we became pregnant, we may never have thought about the mystery of life. But now that a tiny, unknown being is forming inside us, we have sort of come right up against the ultimate mystery. It makes us pause and think about the larger questions: "How can my body create new life?" "Do my thoughts and feelings impact my baby?" "Does he already know who I am?" "Who is he?" These are questions that can never be completely answered, but pondering them connects us to something larger than ourselves.

When I experience the mystery unfolding within me, I realize that it is all around me as well. It is the source of all things beautiful.

Certainly, I wouldn't pretend not to need the electronic accoutrements of modern life, yet one thing is clear: I need time away from the beeps, bells, and buzzes.

🐾 EVELYN RICHARDS

*E*xpectant mothers need time away from the electronic devices that fill our lives: the rings of the telephone, radio alarms, and the blare of TV advertisers. It is essential that we restore our souls with simple, quiet pleasures such as arranging a bouquet of flowers, soaking in a perfumed bath, strolling through antique shops, browsing in a card store, or sipping tea while composing a letter. These quiet, solitary activities will rejuvenate us and help us to pull away from some of the static and jarring noises of modern life.

I may live in the electronic age, but I need not inhabit it every moment of my day.

*A mother's joy begins when new life is stirring inside,
a tiny heartbeat is heard, and a flutter of kicks
reminds her that she is never alone.*

♪ CAROLINE JOYCE

*M*onths before anyone notices, we are aware of the many changes taking place in our body. Our breasts are tender and sore, our waist thickens, and we are more prone to blemishes. We are so proud to be pregnant that we can't wait for our belly to announce it to the world. We stroke our blooming belly, hoping others will notice that "something is different about us." We wear fuller dresses, wishing they'd suspect. Little by little our secret pops out. Until one day we strut around like a proud peacock with our body's pronouncement: "I'm going to be a mother!"

During the first trimester I will have to announce my pregnancy myself if I want to share the good news with others.

*Someday after we have mastered the winds, the
waves, the tides and gravity, we shall harness for
God the energies of love. Then for the second time in
the history of the world, man will have discovered
fire.*

❀ PIERRE TEILHARD DE CHARDIN

*L*ove is a powerful force. And if we have not
fully experienced it before, we will feel its
consuming fire within a few short months. Even
during pregnancy, we get glimpses of it as we find
ourselves hopelessly falling in love with a person
we have never even seen. Once our baby issues
forth from our body, we will be overwhelmed by
the love we feel—now if we can just harness that
love . . .

**The heat of love is a fire that does not burn. It
warms my very soul.**

If there is magic on this planet, it is contained in water.

🦶 LOREN EISELEY

All of us have watery beginnings. We slosh inside our mother's womb, content in the warm, rocking motion of our fluid home. We think of our baby gently swaying back and forth, hearing the steady beat of our heart, while immersed in fluid and soothing darkness.

All of us wish we could return to that magical place now and again. When we're in need of a cozy womb we can curl up on the softest sofa in the house and wrap ourselves in a cuddly blanket. But since the best wombs contain water, a long soak submerged in the bathtub is the best way to feel weightless and buoyant.

I am a creature of the water, returning again and again to my earliest memories of magic.

My fullest concentration of energy is available to me when I integrate all the parts of who I am, opening, allowing power from particular sources of my being to flow back and forth freely without restrictions or externally imposed definitions.

♫ AUDRE LORDE

*P*regnancy opens us to other parts of our being which, until now, may have been dormant or hidden away. We will find out that no matter how many baby books we read, we are the ultimate authority: it is up to us to navigate the challenges and make the best decisions for our child. Every day we will have to make decisions on our child's behalf that will stretch us beyond the person we thought we were—whether it's choosing the best mom-and-baby class, dealing with colic, or researching the side effects of immunizations. And we'll discover new aspects of ourselves to draw on.

Motherhood will give me the opportunity to know myself, more fully, as a multidimensional woman.

Nothing is worth more than this day.

      ❦ EDITH WHARTON

*E*ver had a perfect day where nothing goes wrong? You feel loved and cherished? All is right with the world? Think about that day. Then think about creating a perfect day for yourself. Is there a day spa you can check into? A café with overstuffed chairs where you can curl up and read magazines while it storms outside? A friend you can call to join you for a night out dancing or a walk on the beach?

Allow yourself a day. One perfect day.

To feel completely content for a day is a gift that I can give myself.

Have no friends not equal to yourself.

🐾 CONFUCIUS

*P*regnancy often brings changes to our friendships. Our single friends may become frustrated by our unavailability, and for a time, the offers to go out may dwindle down to nothing. Those friends who have already crossed the threshold into motherhood may become closer now that we share a common life passage. And those friends who drain us by always taking and rarely returning the favor may fall away as our time becomes more limited and valuable.

With motherhood comes a natural sorting process. My true friends will withstand the changing phases of my life.

Learning is not attained by chance, it must be sought with ardor and attended to with diligence.

♫ ABIGAIL ADAMS

There's a reason why we expectant mothers read so voraciously. We are attending to our learning; we are preparing for our new job as "mother." The truth is, parenting does not come completely naturally to most of us. It is far more difficult and demanding than we could have imagined, and the more we know about it ahead of time, the better off we'll be.

I will learn all I can before my baby's birth, knowing there will be much more to learn in the years to come.

Hope is the feeling you have that the feeling you have isn't permanent.

🌸 JEAN KERR

et's face it, most of the fears and anxieties about becoming a mother can be handled with the help of close friends, mothers' groups, family members, physicians, and parenting books. However, when we can't seem to shake a difficult feeling for a period of time, we might want to consider the help of a professional counselor. Perhaps we have fears about being a good mother that are related to our own past. Or we've been plagued with troubling thoughts about giving birth and they just don't seem to go away. If we reach out for help, we can overcome our fears and anxieties and feel hope again.

I may need a professional to remind me that my feelings aren't permanent. I will ask for help if I need it.

These impossible women! How they do get around us! The poet was right: can't live with them, or without them!

👣 ARISTOPHANES

*H*ow many of us had to talk our husbands into having *just one more child*? Our maternal instincts kicked in and we longed for "one more" or we wanted to try one more time for a girl. In some cases, the clock was ticking and we wanted to have that last child, or our first child, before it was too late. Whatever the reason, our husbands probably knew they didn't stand a chance.

The desire to have a baby can be so strong. It defies rationality.

A little girl, asked where her home was, replied,
"where mother is."

♪ KEITH L. BROOKS

*I*sn't it wonderful to return home when you're pregnant? Usually, our mothers are waiting with open arms to be a part of the experience. They share in our excitement and talk about our own birth in awed tones: "I couldn't believe how beautiful you were when I first laid eyes on you." "You were so precious. You had a head of black hair that stood straight up." They want to help us buy baby blankets, booties, pacifiers, sleepers, and car seats. They want to be close to us during this special time so they can share our journey into motherhood and reexperience their own.

Pregnancy gives me the opportunity to reconnect to my mother in a new and profound way. We will come home to each other.

I'm tired of all this nonsense about beauty being only skin-deep. That's deep enough.

🌸 JEAN KERR

*H*ow many of us have attempted to look sexy during the final months of pregnancy only to find that our maternity clothes make us look more like an ostrich than a peacock? It's the strangest thing about pregnancy. On the one hand, our voluptuous breasts and tummies appear to be luminous and exquisite like a full harvest moon. On the other hand, it doesn't take much to cross the line into the ridiculous and to look more like a cow on stilts than a fertility goddess.

Perhaps if I want to look sexy during the final months of my pregnancy, I'd have better success walking around the house in the nude.

Why is it that fools always have the instinct to hunt out the unpleasant secrets of life, and the hardiness to mention them?

🦶 EMILY EDEN

*P*eople can be so foolish around expectant mothers. They relate the most horrible birth-gone-wrong stories in our presence. They gossip about husbands who strayed because their wives were too busy with the new baby. They lament the fact that their youth was stolen by the demands of motherhood, failing to mention the fact that they smoked, lived on fried foods, and rarely exercised.

When we find ourselves around people like this, it's best not to worry about the tales they are spinning and whether they are true. Rather, we must ask ourselves whether we are in danger of becoming infected by their negativity, and if so, we should seek out more positive company.

Foolish is as foolish does. I'd do best not to subject myself to the fools of the world.

He had but one eye, and the popular prejudice runs in favor of two.

♫ CHARLES DICKENS

*W*e live in a time when society's ideal of beauty is limited to a select few. While some of our children may match these commercial images of what is attractive, most of our children will not. It is up to us, then, to encourage our child to see his or her own, unique beauty. The beauty that is reflected in our eyes, not on the television screen.

I will teach my children to be happy with the beauty they possess instead of trying to measure up to external images.

Though boys throw stones at frogs in sport, the frogs do not die in sport, but in earnest.

🌸 BION

As we move into motherhood many of us are rethinking the issue of child rearing. We want to raise boys who are thoughtful, considerate, and sensitive to people and animals. We also want them to know how to succeed in the world. By the same token, we want to raise girls who are compassionate, mindful, and respectful of all living creatures. We also want them to excel.

Not so long ago, gender roles heavily influenced the choices available to our children. Luckily, today, our children's horizons are broader. They have more options. They can simply be good, sensitive, and powerful people.

I want my children to be the kind of people who value life. It is up to me to teach them the values I believe in.

First ponder, then dare.

HELMUTH VON MOLTKE

*P*revious generations viewed pregnancy as a delicate condition whereby women were considered virtually incapacitated. Today, this is no longer the case. Except perhaps on health insurance forms, where pregnancy leave is synonymous with disability leave, pregnant women are anything but disabled. We continue to hike, bike, ride rivers, chair meetings, wrestle with children on the playground, walk the dogs, rock climb, dance, track animals in the bush, make love, and run a busy household. Incapacitated? I don't think so!

Unless my physician tells me otherwise, I will continue to live my life to the fullest during my pregnancy.

I always knew when your mama had them hot flashes. She'd flutter her fan faster than a humming-bird's wings.

♫ WILLENE WILLAFRED

W hile I was with child my body would some-times become so hot that I wanted to jump out of my skin. It was as though my son radiated warmth straight from the womb, as if I were carry-ing a little heater inside that would elevate my tem-perature at a moment's notice. My face would flush; I would sweat; my thirst couldn't be quenched.

The only way to escape the intense heat was to jump into a cold bath or the local pool and watch the steam rise off my body.

When you're hot, you're hot. Pregnancy is one of those times.

*If I know a song of Africa . . . does Africa know a
song of me?*

                      ❀ ISAK DINESEN

*E*very one of us has a special place where
treasured memories were made. Sometimes
we have to travel far to return there. Other times,
we need only step out of our back door and it is as
though we have been transported back in time.
Think about it. Is there a special place you hold
dear? Do you call it home? Perhaps, while nesting
during pregnancy, you could create an atmosphere
reminiscent of your special place, a place that
brings contentment and comfort. When your infant
arrives you can feed him, rock him, and sing to him
in this place, and before long, it will become a special memory for both of you.

**I will draw from the treasured memories of my
past to create a special place where my child and
I can be at home.**

The vigorous, the healthy, and the happy survive and multiply.

🐾 CHARLES DARWIN

ot every large family is like the Waltons. Those of us who were one child among many know the problems inherent in families that multiply. Often there was not enough attention to go around, not enough money to go around, and, unfortunately, sometimes, not enough love to go around. Luckily, today, pregnancy and family size is an option. We can choose to have only one child if that is fitting. Or if we enjoy children and a noisy, bustling household, we can have a small army either by birthing our own, adopting, or a combination thereof. If we decide on our family size based on our own values and financial means, we stand a better chance of being happy with our choice.

I will choose the number of children I want, trusting what is right for me and my family.

Go to your bosom: Knock there, and ask your heart what it doth know.

♪ WILLIAM SHAKESPEARE

All of us have strengths. We have weaknesses. However, when we decide ahead of time, either consciously or unconsciously, that our soon-to-be-born child will make up for our shortcomings, we do him a grave injustice. Chances are, instead of encouraging him to pursue those passions and interests he is attracted to, we will tend to steer him toward our favorite pastimes. Instead of allowing him to follow his heart, we will force him to master the pursuits we deem of value. The result: he will think we want a clone of our ideal self instead of someone like him.

I will share my interests with my child while helping him to discover his own.

Reading to Baby

Some books are to be tasted, others to be swallowed, and some few to be chewed and digested.

🌸 SIR FRANCIS BACON

Isn't it wonderful to read our favorite books to our tummy? Before our baby is born, we are sharing some of our most cherished stories and retelling adventures of days gone by. Not only that, but we are helping our infant to become accustomed to our voice and to absorb the words and rhythms of great poets, historical figures, and wise women. Even if it turns out that our child doesn't share our literary tastes once outside the womb, for now, we have a captive audience.

I will savor my favorite books with my baby-to-be and look forward to the time when he can turn the pages with me.

Write injuries in sand, kindnesses in marble.

FRENCH PROVERB

*U*nfortunately, it is all too easy to allow others' transgressions to build resentment. Mom didn't fly out for the birth as she had promised. It's been three months since the birth of our child, and Dad has yet to see her.

While incidents like these are hurtful, if we hold a grudge, it only causes us more pain. Perhaps we can be more realistic about the type of parents we have. They may not be the classic grandparents we see in the movies, always anticipating their children's needs, always available and ready to lend a helping hand. Our parents might have different things to offer. If we focus on the kindnesses they do show instead of on their inconsiderate and occasionally unfair behavior, we can forgive them more easily, and enjoy them more when they are around.

My parents' thoughtless actions can hurt. I must lower my expectations and learn to focus on and appreciate the good things they do for my child.

The optimist proclaims that we live in the best of all possible worlds; and the pessimist fears this is true.

♫ JAMES BRANCH CABELL

*A*s expectant mothers we can't avoid looking at the state of the world and wondering what we are bringing our children into. Countries are at war. Famines plague the earth. Gang violence is no longer an isolated, urban phenomenon. The earth's resources are being destroyed and consumed at an incredible rate. The list is endless.

At times, it's difficult to be genuinely optimistic. Yet the fact that we still believe it is good to bring a child into the world illustrates the depth of our faith in humanity. Our doubts will not win out.

I carry optimism in my heart. My child will feel the depth of my faith.

Between two evils, I always pick the one I never tried before.

🌸 MAE WEST

*E*ating chocolate or drinking an espresso can feel like the most delicious sin when we have been eating nothing but free-range chicken, organic vegetables, and fresh fruit during our pregnancy. While we should be proud of ourselves for being such good girls and regularly avoiding sugary, unhealthy foods, it can't hurt to splurge on something sinful once in a while. How about picking out something we've never tried before?

Even good girls need to be bad once in a while. Today is as good a day as any!

Who's on first, What's on second, I Don't Know's on third—

🦶 BUD ABBOTT AND LOU COSTELLO

*T*rying to nail down all the details related to pregnancy and childbirth can be confusing. "When do I go in for my first blood test?" "Now, what did the doctor tell me about folic acid?" we ask ourselves. "And what was the name of the birthing coach my friend recommended?" At times we feel like we're in an Abbott and Costello comedy act, and for the life of us, we can't remember who's on first or third.

Keeping track of all the details concerning my pregnancy can be difficult. It helps if I keep a sense of humor *and* a notebook.

Confidence

Challenge is a dragon with a gift in its mouth. . . .
Tame the dragon and the gift is yours.

♫ NOELA EVANS

*P*regnancy can present us with all kinds of challenges. Perhaps we are diabetic and must carefully monitor our blood sugar in order to carry our pregnancy to term. Maybe we are anemic and must respect our body's need for more iron and a less strenuous workout regime. If we have a history of miscarriage, it takes courage to try "one more time." Whenever we are challenged by the twists and turns pregnancy can take, we are given the opportunity to "tame the dragon" and feel the gift of confidence that comes with seeing a difficult situation through.

When I befriend the dragon, I feel more confident.

A difference of taste in jokes is a great strain on the affections.

⚓ GEORGE ELIOT

*R*arely, when a woman is pregnant, are fat jokes appreciated. Sure, our partner may think he's helping us "lighten up" by getting us to laugh at ourselves, but his timing is off. He might think he's distracting us from our weight gain when, in actuality, he's calling attention to it.

Before we contemplate divorce, it would be a good idea to tactfully mention our different taste in humor. He may not be aware of the fact that his "fat" jokes make us feel bad and put a strain on our affections.

My partner's jokes could be his awkward way of trying to make light of things. I will laugh when I can and ask him to change his stand-up routine when necessary.

. . . in the pulse that repeats the pulse of my own veins and in the breath that mingles with my breath. Now my belly is as noble as my heart.

GABRIELA MISTRAL

If we open ourselves, pregnancy can provide us with the experience of being completely in tune with another human being. Even in utero, our little one is communicating with us. We can feel the flutters of movement like Morse code tapping out messages we can understand only when we listen with our hearts. In Kenya, for example, it is common for a woman to intuit the temperament of her child long before she is born. And Tibetans think it normal for a pregnant woman to know any past life associations she and her child have had.

If I listen with an intuitive ear, I can hear my unborn child's communications. We are one.

. . . parents should present a lot of interesting possibilities and sponsor the child's mind and growth. The kids that are vital are listened to, read to, and taken places. Many kids these days aren't getting an interesting life; they're getting a secondhand, TV life.

♪ MICHAEL COOKINGHAM

We have nine months to think about the type of life that we would like to give our child. Our visions need not be grand, but they should stem from our values. What is important to us? To have a child who is an avid reader? A child who can blend with other cultures? An analytic child who concerns himself with world affairs? Do we want him to know about art and music, sports and car engines? And is it important to us that he treats others with respect? If we remember to include our child in those activities that hold special meaning for us, we will *both* have a life well lived—not a secondhand life.

I will be an involved parent so my child will experience the richness of life firsthand.

*My mother taught me the legends of our people,
taught me of the sun and sky, the moon and stars,
the clouds and storms.*

🌸 GERONIMO

Storytelling is one of the cornerstones of creativity. Even while our child is in utero, we can tell him the stories we were told as children. We can recite the poems of Dylan Thomas, Maya Angelou, or David Whyte. We can pluck our favorite passages out of books and read them aloud. It doesn't matter how sophisticated the material is or how simple. If it inspires us, moves us, fills our hearts with glee, our baby will love the sound of our words and thrill to it, too.

Native peoples know the value of storytelling. Sharing *my* favorite legends and stories with my child will expand his vision and knowledge of the world, even before he is born.

April,
Comes like an idiot, babbling, and strewing flowers.

🦶 EDNA ST. VINCENT MILLAY

Spring infuses us with its silly joy. "There's nothing like having a baby in springtime," a mother of four once told me. "I'm always happier, more active, more ready to laugh." And it's true: as winter thaws, spring wakes us up, invigorating us with its blooming flowers, warm breezes, and bright skies. Although our size has increased and our bodies feel cumbersome, we have blossomed like spring buds—full of the season's green and giddy promise.

Spring is like no other season. My baby and I will enjoy its offerings.

Speak to the earth, and it shall teach thee.

♫JOB 12:8

*P*regnancy can awaken us to the pulse of the planet. Sometimes we even experience the collective beat of the human heart. When others are sad and distraught, we feel it. When conflict is present, we sense it. When genuine joy infuses some of the faces we greet on our way to the subway, we know it. If we listen, we will hear the many voices of the earth and her people as they whisper their happiness and sorrow into our ears.

Pregnancy teaches me to be more sensitive to the plights and joys of others.

Whoever takes the child by the hand takes the mother by the heart.

☘ ENGLISH PROVERB

*I*t's easy to think we will want to spend every waking moment with our infant once he is born. But the fact is, we will need time to ourselves. If we've had a C-section, we will need lots of rest to recover from surgery. If our baby is a voracious eater, we will need nutritious meals and plenty of sleep to produce enough milk. And naps are a must.

Although our child's birth may seem far away, it's not too soon to line up help. Put out the word in the neighborhood. Post signs at your local YMCA or Jewish community center: "Baby-sitter Wanted." Accumulate a list of available teenagers who are trustworthy and reliable.

If I begin the search now, I will have a better chance of finding help when I need it most.

We cannot be a source of strength unless we nurture our own strength.

🦶 M. SCOTT PECK

As women, we possess a strength and vitality that our family often draws upon. Yet when we are pregnant, we often need to gather our inner resources for ourselves and our unborn child. We know that these resources are not without limits and now is not the time to stretch ourselves *to* the limit.

Pregnancy can be an important time to learn how best to rejuvenate our body, mind, and spirit whether through meditation, exercise, play, or any activity that brings us inner peace. After all, there's a little one on the way who, like the other members of our family, will depend on us as a source of strength.

As a mother, I must always be on the lookout for ways to nurture and increase my strength.

Few of us, I learned, are really "born" for the job of motherhood. Rather, being a good mother is a privilege earned through hard work and a continual, daily recommitment to the importance of the work. It means being willing to confront the very worst in ourselves, and brave enough not to run away from it when the going gets rough.

♫ LINDA BURTON

I've often heard it said: "Motherhood is the toughest job you'll ever love." Isn't it surprising, then, when we discover after a month at home with our infant that we don't want to go back to work? Sure, we had everything planned out. Three months of maternity leave, place Baby in a daycare facility, and return to work. Yet as the weeks passed, we felt our heart sink at the thought of being away from our little one. We weren't comfortable with the idea of having someone else raise our child. We wanted to do it ourselves, every day, no matter how daunting the challenges.

If I change my mind about staying home once my baby is born, I may have to do some quick thinking. Perhaps I should consider it now as an option.

Making the decision to have a child is momentous. It is to decide forever to have your heart go walking around outside your body.

🌺 ELIZABETH STONE

*H*ow inexplicable is the beauty of love we feel when our infant suddenly flutters within us. We are carrying another life inside, protecting and nourishing it with our body and our heart. If we become consumed with meetings at work, visiting relatives, or remodeling a room before the baby arrives, one heavy thump in our womb is like a knock on the door, reminding us where our heart is. And we reply: "I am with you. I am here. I love you, little one."

There is no love more beautiful than a mother's love for her child.

We need another brother. This one spits out his food and is disgusting. The other new one will be better.

🦶 JASON BROOKS

*I*sn't it funny how older siblings view their younger counterparts? Though there are precious moments when they are the perfect "big brother" or "big sister," many of them think that returning a "faulty model" to the hospital is an available option. What they don't realize is that they, too, spit up on their clothes, pooped in strange colors, stuffed gross objects into their mouths, and vomited halfway across the room. We need to help them welcome this strange, sweet—and yes, sometimes disgusting—new creature into the fold.

A new baby may be a mixed blessing for my other children. I will be there to help them meet the challenge and maybe even enjoy it.

I was a gallbladder attack.

♫ CARLA CLAUSSEN

Sometimes we discover we're pregnant in the most unexpected ways. We might think we are "just getting fat" until our annual checkup reveals another cause for our weight gain. Or we complain to our physician that we feel nauseated, tired and have trouble focusing and she casually asks, "Is there any way you could be pregnant?" Or perhaps we have been trying to conceive without success, and once we have given up, it happens. We mistake our symptoms for indigestion until it is obvious that our period will be nine months "late."

It didn't matter how I found out I was pregnant, it was such good news!

God will be present whether asked or not.

                🌺 LATIN PROVERB

On the delivery table we will most likely be concentrating on our husband's coaching and soothing words, the nurse's attentiveness to our needs, and our doctor's directives. As labor intensifies, we probably won't think about who else is present for our child's birth. But, be assured, God and the angels wouldn't miss it!

En route to the hospital I will say a silent prayer to the guardian angel who welcomes every child into the world.

Bed Rest

A friend in need is a friend indeed.

🦶 PROVERB

*P*rescribed bed rest during pregnancy can be a drag. Accustomed to an active lifestyle, we get grumpy watching television. We can read only so many books, and we're sure we can hear our muscles dissolving into fatty tissue. Although we agree to do whatever's necessary to prevent a premature birth, being perpetually horizontal can be very confining.

Isn't it heavenly when a girlfriend who recently graduated from massage school drops by with her portable table, lights a few candles, and relaxes our stiff back with jasmine and ylang-ylang oil? Or another friend comes by and brings us a video? Friendly gestures such as these make bed rest more bearable.

I am grateful for the friends who can anticipate my needs without my having to ask.

I am my mother's daughter . . . and although it's been twenty years since I left home, her sayings form a perpetual long-playing record on my inner-ear turntable.

♫ CAROL SHIELDS

For good or ill, we are a lot like our mothers and we instinctively model our own mothering on theirs. As we mature, we come to appreciate our mothers' finest attributes and the ways in which they've shaped our lives. Although we will not be identical in our mothering, we can draw on our many—or few—fond memories to answer the question "What would Mom have done in this situation?" And we can either follow suit or do the direct opposite!

My mother is forever a part of me. I will nurture the best parts of her within myself and learn from her mistakes.

It occurs to me over and over that I am much too self-centered, cynical, eccentric, and edgy to raise a baby, especially alone.

❦ ANNE LAMOTT

Raising a child single-handedly is an act of courage, though it may sometimes feel more like stupidity. Either way, it takes enormous strength and endurance to figure out how to juggle the day-to-day demands. Unlike other mothers, who can ask for assistance from their mates, we must rely on ourselves to do what may seem impossible—alone. That doesn't mean it *is* impossible.

Fortunately, there are a lot of us out there. We can draw strength and wisdom from each other, and share advice, favors, laughter, and tears. And we can accept the help of friends and family, too. Let's face it, we have to!

Overwhelming as the challenges may be from time to time, especially for a single mom, I know that I can do it. I will look to my peers for encouragement and ask for help when I need it.

Take your life into your own hands and what happens? A terrible thing: no one to blame.

🦶 ERICA JONG

Taking responsibility for our lives is, at first, not much fun. When things go wrong, we have to look to ourselves to fix them. When our words wound another, it is up to us to make amends. If a check bounces,we have to rectify the situation. Of course, we can always try to convince ourselves that it was our friend's fault or the bank's fault, or that it isn't our job to fix things. But, if we do that, we will be a child raising a child. It's time to grow up!

Someone said: "The truth will set you free, but first it will make you miserable." I will let myself know what is true even if it means I have to take full responsibility for myself and my actions.

*In the middle of the journey of our life I came to
myself within a dark wood where the straight way
was lost.*

♫ DANTE ALIGHIERI

W e can move along on a set course, expecting everything to go as planned, only to
wake up one morning and discover that something
profound has changed. Our marriage may be falter-
ing, we may not want to return to the same unfulfilling job, an exciting new company may offer us a
promotion in a different part of the country, or there
may be a death in the family. Suddenly, we are
presented with options that we have never considered. And, as if having a baby wasn't change
enough, we uproot our lives and take a leap of faith
in a new direction.

**I might not always welcome the unexpected
twists and turns of life, but I will be thankful for
the new opportunities they present to me and
my family.**

Throughout my pregnancy I lived in constant dread of delivery. . . . I was concerned about two things: that whatever it was that was growing and wiggling in my belly could not be human; and that it would never come out. . . .

🌹 CELINA SPIEGEL

*F*or some of us, the process of giving birth seems almost impossible. Our low threshold of pain, lack of endurance, and fear have convinced us that we'll have to be unconscious on the delivery table in order to get this baby out. But the truth is, millions of women have gone through birth before us, and millions will go after us. Birth may not be easy, but women have done it since the beginning of time—and we can, too.

That said, while some hold natural childbirth to be the only good childbirth, modern medicine has given us many more choices and a much greater chance of a safe and successful delivery. So, whatever our personal desires for labor and delivery, the most important goal to keep in mind is this: a healthy baby and a healthy mom.

Like The Little Engine That Could, I won't give up. My daily mantra will be "I think I can, I think I can, I think I can . . ." And I know I will!

Heroism . . . is endurance for one moment more.

🦶 GEORGE KENNAN

Never is this saying more true than during labor. Just when we fear we might not have an ounce of strength left, we endure another set of contractions. When we think we are too exhausted to push anymore, we take a deep breath and rise to the occasion. If we have a moment when we think we're doing a bad job, we receive a smile from our mate and we're back on track. We hold on for just one more moment, one moment more, one more again, and eventually our baby is born.

Just one more contraction, one more push, one more, one more. . . . I will birth my baby moment by moment with the endurance of a true hero.

It is a wise father that knows his own child.

♫ WILLIAM SHAKESPEARE

Having a partner who is fully engaged in parenthood is an enormous gift. He gets just as excited as we do when the baby kicks. He puts his ear to our stomach and listens for sounds we cannot possibly hear. He talks to our baby and plays guitar for him in utero. He begins relating to his child and sharing who he is before they have officially met. Watching him, we feel confident that he will play an active role with our child for the rest of their lives.

An involved father is a loving father. I will do whatever I can to include my partner equally in the joys and challenges of parenting.

*The events in our lives happen in a sequence in time,
but in their significance to ourselves, they find their
own order . . . the continuous thread of revelation.*

🌺 EUDORA WELTY

*P*erhaps this pregnancy holds a special significance in our lives. If we have given a
previous child up for adoption because we were
too young to raise her, this pregnancy may mean a
second chance at motherhood. If our lives used to
be chaotic and alcohol was a problem, we can now
birth a baby as a healthy, drug-free mother. If we
have lost other children in miscarriages, being pregnant now allows us to put away any remaining
grief. Whatever our pregnancy's significance, we
will know its order in our lives.

**Pregnancy can be significant in so many ways. I
will allow it to heal old wounds, bring closure to
previous events, and help me to open to the next
phase of my life.**

If you do not want to know the sex of your child until birth, write "DO NOT WANT TO KNOW THE SEX" on a name label and adhere it to the lab paperwork. If you have to, stick extra labels on the forehead of any lab technician you suspect might inadvertently let your little secret slip out.

🐾 MILDRED BIXBY, R.N.

*D*eciding whether to find out Baby's sex before the birth is a big decision for many couples. Rarely do parents have a casual opinion about the matter. They either want to know or they don't. If you and your husband strongly prefer not to know whether you're having a boy or a girl, you'd better make it crystal clear to everyone in the doctor's office and in the hospital. Otherwise, one little slip of the tongue can ruin your surprise.

"Loose lips sink ships," and, sometimes, eager hearts. My husband and I had better team up and tell everyone that we prefer *not* to know the sex of our child until its birth.

The bluebird carries the sky on his back.

♫ HENRY DAVID THOREAU

*E*ver see a pregnant woman dance? Pedal a
bicycle on a country road? Rock bareback
on a cantering horse? She is like the bluebird, unfet-
tered, unencumbered by her size, effortlessly carrying the sky on her back. She is beauty personified.

**I will enjoy the times during pregnancy when I
feel spontaneous, voluptuous, and vibrant.**

My energy goes through phases just like the moon.
🌸 DARYN STIER

Certain phases of pregnancy can make us feel lethargic and lazy. Like couch potatoes, we don't want to exert ourselves any more than we absolutely have to. We hate work. We hate the pressure. We hate the routine. Then, just when we think we'll never have any energy again, we wake up, ready to take on new projects, complete old ones, and prepare the nursery all at the same time! A few weeks later, we feel sluggish again and wish our mate would peel grapes and feed us by hand instead of expecting dinner on the table by six o'clock. Such is the ebb and flow of our bodies!

If I follow my body's cues I will know when to keep an executive's pace and when to sip lemonade in the shade.

Never doubt that a small group of thoughtful, committed citizens can change the world; indeed, it is the only thing that ever does.

🐾 MARGARET MEAD

*H*ave you ever seen a group of mothers who are tired of drivers speeding through the neighborhood? When they join together to lobby the city for additional speed bumps, they are quite effective. And what about the group of mothers who decided to lobby for tougher penalties for drunk drivers? They changed federal laws about driving while intoxicated and held careless individuals responsible for their actions. No small task.

The transition into motherhood often makes us aware of how vital it is to protect those we love and can spur us into unexpected activism. Even for those of us who are shy or timid, or see ourselves as "not the kind of woman who becomes politically active," pregnancy can change all that.

The process of becoming a mother is changing more than my body. It is bringing a new awareness of what it means to take care of those I love—sometimes in dramatic ways.

Itchy abdomen, hemorrhoids, headaches, nasal congestion, absentmindedness, swelling of the ankles, backache, leg cramps, varicose veins, nosebleeds, fewer mood swings . . .

♫ ARLENE EISENBERG, HEIDI E. MURKOFF, AND
SANDEE E. HATHAWAY

*L*ists like these can make us want to reabsorb our baby, sending her back from where she came. The more we read our pregnancy books, the more we frighten ourselves. We're like medical students who study various diseases only to think they are afflicted by every single one. But the fact is, few of us experience all of these unpleasant symptoms of pregnancy, or at least not all of them at the same time. Even if we do, it is helpful to remember that they are usually short-lived.

It's better to know what to expect when I'm expecting. And then be pleased to discover that I won't have to contend with every symptom.

*I suppose you can't have everything, though my
instinctive response to this sentiment is always
"Why not?"*

⚓ MARGARET HALSEY

*A*round the second or third month of pregnancy, we may go through what I call the
princess phase. We want a new wardrobe because
we can't fit into any of our favorite clothes. We want
to eat out every night rather than having to cook.
We want our nails done and our calves massaged.
We want compliments, attention, special treatment,
and the room temperature to be just so. In short,
we're having a princess attack!

**A princess attack will make me temporarily
unbearable. Hopefully, a little pampering will
help me to be less demanding.**

So far today, God, I've done all right. I haven't gossiped, lost my temper; haven't been grumpy, nasty or selfish. I'm really glad of that. But in a few minutes, God, I'm going to get out of bed, and from this point on, I'm going to need a lot of help.

ANONYMOUS

*E*ver gone through a phase when you just don't feel like yourself? You're too tired to mind your manners and too tired to care. Your moods go from sour to extremely sour in a matter of minutes and you think only divine intervention will save you from yourself. As expectant mothers we can lose our charm when we're overly fatigued. We lose our patience after days of back pain and other bodily discomforts, and we lose our smile when plagued with nausea. We wonder if we'll ever feel like our old selves again. In time, we will. In the meantime, we can ask for help.

Praying during the rocky parts of pregnancy is often the best thing I can do for myself. Sometimes it's the *only* thing I can do.

If you were born lucky, even your rooster will lay eggs.

♫ RUSSIAN PROVERB

*L*uck just seems to follow some women around. They decide to get pregnant and—poof—the next month they are. Others try and try to get pregnant without any success. In fact, it can become so frustrating that they give up the idea of bearing their own children and seek out adoption options. Luckily, there are many options for those of us who may not be so lucky when it comes to fertility. We can adopt, receive infertility treatments, or just keep trying. In most cases, we will prevail and have a child we can call our own.

Sometimes it takes more than luck to have a successful pregnancy. If I need to, I will pursue new options.

Beware all enterprises that require new clothes.
        ❦ HENRY DAVID THOREAU

*P*regnancy is an enterprise that definitely requires new clothes. Maternity outfits are now chic and stylish, tailored and professional, flattering and colorful. Pregnant women can be both fashionable *and* comfortable simultaneously. The only drawback is that maternity clothes can be expensive. We would do well to remember that our new wardrobe need only clothe us for nine months. And often friends are happy to lend us a pregnancy outfit for a special occasion.

Being pregnant no longer means that I have to "dress down" or look dowdy. I will wear the latest maternity fashions with panache.

Encouragement

Mama exhorted her children at every opportunity to "jump at de sun." We might not land on the sun, but at least we would get off the ground.

> ZORA NEALE HURSTON

Somewhere around the second trimester we begin encouraging our child. When she does somersaults in our belly, we pat our belly and just have to tell the nearest person, as though no one else's child has ever done such a thing. After her birth, we will keep it up—encouraging her to sit up, crawl, walk, and, eventually, tie her shoes. We want her to know we are always behind her.

Encouraging my child to "jump at de sun" lets her know that I believe in her. I will take every opportunity to help her soar.

Trust only movement. Life happens on the level of events, not words. Trust movement.

♫ ALFRED ADLER

*I*t's not enough to say that we are going to take good care of ourselves during pregnancy, we must do it. If the stress of a miserable job is overwhelming us, then we must look into alternatives: short-term disability leave, a sabbatical, bed rest, or dipping into a savings account for a few months. If we still consume alcohol or smoke cigarettes, we need to stop NOW until after the baby is born. If we aren't pampering ourselves on occasion, it might be time to dip into a warm, scented bath, get a facial, or have a friend or a sister brush and style our hair the way we used to when we were kids. Talking won't do, we need to move and take action.

I will take action today.

Heaven is the place where the donkey finally catches up with his carrot: hell is the eternity while he waits for it.

🌸 RUSSELL GREEN

*D*uring our second or third pregnancy, patience may not be one of our virtues. We might want to skip the pregnancy to get on with the task of raising our next child. Instead of the in utero experience feeling special, it becomes one more inconvenience we must endure. Nine months seem like an eternity.

While we can't reduce the gestation period, we can find creative ways to make the time go more quickly. We can focus on other things: playing with our children, planning special events, inviting friends over for a potluck, driving up to the city to take in an opera, getting lost in a good book when the baby-sitter is on duty, and focusing on daily tasks and projects. Before we know it, we'll be so busy with our new baby, pregnancy will seem like a distant memory.

Involving myself in the activities of life makes the time go more quickly.

Sex itself must always, it seems to me, come to us as a sacrament and be so used, or it is meaningless.
🐾 MAY SARTON

*I*t is far too easy these days to rush through our lives as though on fast-forward. We forget to savor the precious moments. Fortunately, pregnancy offers us the opportunity to be more in touch with those things that hold special meaning to us, like being close to our partner. We can feel a different dimension in our love for each other since bringing a new life into the world. And we can make time to embrace each other and experience the sacredness of the union that brought our baby into our lives.

Life has offered me the most sacred blessings. I am thankful.

We are all being called into our own greatness. . . .
♪ JEAN HOUSTON

*P*regnancy is a call into our own greatness. In the upcoming months, our strengths will be called into action, our patience will be tried, and we will learn more than we ever could have imagined about our limits as well as our ability to surpass them. While we may try to incorporate our pregnancy into our day-to-day lives as though little has changed, we soon discover that *everything has changed*—even if our lives appear to be the same on the outside.

I have answered the call. Life will never be the same.

Breaking wedding vows breaks hearts, no matter how many reasons we repeat to ourselves.

⚓ ELLEN SUE STERN

*O*ccasionally marriages fail at the most inopportune time: like when we have a baby on the way. The pain is awful. Whether we initiated the breakup or not, we feel betrayed. The promises we made to each other on our wedding day were not strong enough to hold, and we find ourselves advancing into unknown territory: a future as a single mother that we had never intended. Now not only will we have to prepare for the birth alone, but we will have to redirect our focus and begin to accept the fact that we may be raising our child between two households or all by ourselves. It's not easy, and it's not fair—but there's no turning back. We just have to do the very best we can in difficult circumstances.

"Stuff happens," and it happens to good people. I must be resilient in the face of unexpected and devastating change.

What age is best for a woman to have children?
Physically, in her twenties; emotionally, in her
thirties; financially, in her forties.

🦶 JULIE TILSNER

*I*sn't it wonderful that women are having
babies at later and later ages? Supermodel
Cheryl Tiegs recently had twin boys at age fifty-two!
Technology and healthier living has pushed back
the time button on our biological clocks, so that age
is no longer the primary factor about when we
become pregnant. With this new freedom, we can
become mothers when the time is right for us.

**I need not fear the number of my years. Every
age has its benefits.**

Expect nothing. Live frugally. On surprise.
♬ ALICE WALKER

*L*ike it or not, grandparents have preferences. Most grandpas want a grandson and most grandmas want a granddaughter. They imagine an instant bond based on gender, and forget about the possibility that their grandchild may have nothing in common with them. "When my grandson arrives, he'll be my first mate," our father informs us. "I'll take her to the spa for a girls' night out," our mother tells us. Won't they be surprised. . . .

My parents might have expectations about their grandchild. Hopefully, they can set these aside and welcome my baby unconditionally into their lives.

*. . . everything grows rounder and wider and
weirder, and I sit in the middle of it all and wonder
who in the world you will turn out to be.*

❧ CARRIE FISHER

*T*o pretend this is simply another event is to
deny ourselves the wonderful privilege and
the wondrous amazement of being pregnant. It's
also the only time in our child's life that we will be
free to fantasize about who and what this child will
be like. For once she is born, the dream-child we
envisioned will be replaced by a real child—even
more wonderful than we could have imagined, but
also different in many ways. So why not take the
time now to contemplate our navels—that is, if we
can still find our navels!—and reflect on the weird-
ness and wonder of it all.

**I will sit down and allow myself time to simply
be astonished by life.**

Anxiety is the interest paid on trouble before it is due.
♙ WILLIAM INGE

While we're pregnant, all sorts of people will tell us not to worry. Although their intentions are good—they are simply trying to alleviate our anxiety—these words alone will not drive worry from our thoughts: "What if I don't produce enough milk?" "What if my baby can't latch on?" "If breast-feeding is too painful, will I be unable to continue?"

The truth is, it's impossible to predict: some infants refuse to suckle at the breast, while others want to nurse constantly. Luckily, many breast-feeding problems can be difficult but not impossible to resolve with the help of a lactation specialist. Until we have the actual newborn in our arms, we won't know what problems we may encounter or what the best solutions will be.

Asking my midwife or a lactation specialist to talk with me about breast-feeding before the birth is the first step in alleviating my concerns. Learning how best to respond to the needs of my child is the second. Patience is the key.

Grown don't mean nothing to a mother. A child is a child. They get bigger, older, but grown? What's that supposed to mean? In my heart it don't mean a thing.

♫ TONI MORRISON

*I*t is difficult to imagine that one day our child, who is not even born yet, will be an adult. And although he will "be on his own" then, his hardships will still affect us, and his successes will always make us applaud. We will worry about whether he is applying for the right job or dating the right girl or making the right decision, because our lives will be forever intertwined.

When we become pregnant, we really do enter a completely new world, and our lives will never be the same again. As a father of four once said: "Parenting never ends. Not when your child is twenty or forty-five or even sixty. It never ends."

My child is now growing in my heart and there he will always stay.

More children suffer from interference than from non-interference.

🌸 AGATHA CHRISTIE

Sometimes our parents want so desperately to be in on every aspect of the pregnancy and birth that they interfere with our plans. Instead of asking how they can be of help, they tend to take over and run the show. Under these circumstances, it is essential to set limits and be honest about our boundaries. Is our husband comfortable having our mother present during doctor's exams? Do we want our parents in the delivery room for the birth, or would we prefer to call them after the baby arrives? How long do we want them to stay with us after the baby comes home? Explaining our preferences while giving our parents specific tasks helps them feel useful while simultaneously curtailing unwanted interference.

I will find ways to involve my parents that are comfortable for me and my husband.

Body Image

Mirrors should reflect a little more before throwing back images.

🦶 JEAN COCTEAU

*W*e've all heard this complaint: "I never gained this much weight with my first child"—maybe we've even said it ourselves. The truth is, each pregnancy is different. And the fact that we maintained a low weight gain with our first pregnancy doesn't mean we'll be able to do it with our second or third. Our body changes with every one.

I have birthed several children and my body has changed. I may need to accept a new image of myself, one that is voluptuous, womanly, and full.

Bore, n. A person who talks when you wish him to listen.

♪ AMBROSE BIERCE

*I*t isn't enough for an obstetrician to be knowledgeable and experienced. We first-time mothers need to find a doctor with an attentive ear who listens to our questions and answers them to our satisfaction. We want someone we trust who doesn't lecture us about our pregnancy, but, instead, patiently and thoughtfully addresses our concerns. We'll take the time to find a doctor who will make us feel confident and relaxed in his care.

It's important to be selective when choosing a physician or midwife. I want my first experience of birth to be as positive as it can be.

In politics, if you want anything said, ask a man. If you want anything done, ask a woman.

🌸 MARGARET THATCHER

Some of us have husbands who talk about helping out with the kids, yet somehow the help never materializes. We have tried begging, negotiating, even threatening, but to no avail. The status quo remains.

If we are serious about creating change in our family politic, we might have to enlist the help of a therapist in order to move beyond our current dynamic. Long-held attitudes are difficult to change, and while our husband may hear what we're saying, he may need some help understanding what, specifically, we want from him. Having a third party express our needs often leads to better understanding and, eventually, new ways of doing things.

Entrenched habits are hard to change. I may need the help of an outside authority to create a more equitable partnership.

No cord nor cable can so forcibly draw, or hold so fast, as love can do with a twined thread.

ROBERT BURTON

*I*sn't it wonderful when our husbands involve themselves in the pregnancy? They volunteer to sign us up for a local diaper service. They come home with little treasures: teddy bears, rattles, and storybooks. They read the books we've left on the coffee table in order to better understand the birthing process. And they clip articles from the local paper to read to us. We feel loved.

Involving himself in my pregnancy experience is one of the greatest gifts my husband can give me.

I'm a flower, a flower opening and reaching for the sun. You are the sun, Grandma, you are the sun in my life.

♫ KITTY TSUI

Involving grandparents in our children's lives is one of the greatest gifts we can give both of them. Grandparents already know how to handle an infant, change diapers, and sing soothing lullabies. Our little one feels comfortable in their care. And they enjoy helping out with our toddler. They take walks and share secrets, exchange advice and have the time and patience to lend a listening ear. Grandpa's corny jokes are entertaining. Grandma's pecan pie is tradition. Our children sometimes offer our parents a second chance at parenting—one that is more forgiving, flexible, and fun.

My children and I are thankful for my parents' presence in our lives. We will take care of each other throughout the years.

*I always felt that the great high privilege, relief, and
comfort of friendship was that one had to explain
nothing.*

🌸 KATHERINE MANSFIELD

*I*sn't it great to have friends we can say anything to? We can complain about our hemorrhoids, tell them how urine leaks out when we
laugh too hard, and lift up our shirts to show them
our newly acquired stretch marks. Yep, true friends
can share in the nitty-gritty of pregnancy. Chances
are, they can match us word for word with tales of
their own experiences.

**Close friends are comfortable friends. I can say
anything in their presence.**

You can't push the river, you can't change the tide.

🐾 INDIAN PROVERB

Never was this saying more true than in the labor room. If we are in a rush we only frustrate ourselves. We can't make our contractions go any faster. If we try to increase their frequency, we run the risk of our cervix swelling, which would only add time to the delivery. If we become impatient and tense, we can elevate our level of pain and it will seem like days before our baby arrives. Yes, for once in our busy lives, we can't control things by going faster. We must slow down and let the natural process and pace of birth take over.

The birth experience will be more positive for me and everyone involved if I go with the flow instead of rush toward the end.

Don't look back. Something might be gaining on you.
♫ SATCHEL PAIGE

*T*he further along we get in our pregnancy, the better chance our toddler has of catching us. While his legs are growing stronger, we're growing heavier. While his energy is boundless, we can become short of breath. It's a humbling experience. But if we look on the bright side, we realize we're building his confidence without even trying. Besides, it's good practice. Soon he'll have a little brother or sister chasing after *him*.

I delight in being caught by my little man. The odds are in his favor.

Whatever else can be said about sex, it cannot be called a dignified performance.

🌺 HELEN LAWRENSON

Sex during pregnancy can be terribly funny. During our last trimester, we look more like we're doing the Mating-of-the-Water-Buffalo Dance than suave lovers looking sensual. We try closing our eyes to "get into it," but it's no use. The balloon of our belly makes the act of sex look like a circus performance. And the more we try to stifle our giggles, the harder we laugh.

Full-bellied laughter never seemed more apropos!

When you call me that, smile!

🦶 OWEN WISTER

Tempers can flare during pregnancy. Our stomach feels queasy, our energy level is low, older children demand our attention, and we haven't gotten to the gym in over a week. Luckily, humor can take the edge off. Levity helps us regain perspective by laughing at the craziness of our life. Instead of yelling at the kids, try talking out loud to no one in particular and see if they notice. If that doesn't work, have a dialogue with the dog, playing both parts, of course. Our family may think we've lost our marbles, but we know our insanity is temporary—temporary relief.

My sense of humor is a secret weapon to be used when the world overwhelms me.

The soul can split the sky in two and let the face of God shine through.

♫ EDNA ST. VINCENT MILLAY

*M*y grandmother was a talented poet. She also broke horses for a living. One day a spirited stallion bolted into a bucking fit and the saddle horn penetrated her abdomen, rupturing her uterus and ovaries. The doctors told her she would never be able to have children. But not being one to heed the advice of others, she went ahead and got pregnant anyway. Against great odds, my mother was born. Did she say "I told you so"? You bet she did! My grandmother *loved* being right!

Sometimes, in order to have the child I so desire, I must forge a new path; possibly even a dangerous one. I pray the gods will smile on me and my stubborn determination.

A strong woman is a woman determined to do something others are determined not to be done.

🌸 MARGE PIERCY

It takes courage to be a single mother, especially if we have traditional parents who cannot conceive of anyone having a child without a husband. No matter how we try to explain our position, they still cannot accept our choice. Hopefully, after our baby arrives, our parents can set aside their differences and focus on being loving and attentive grandparents.

I must be resolute in my choice to be a single mother, since I will inevitably run up against opposition.

Did you know that women have the greatest chance of becoming pregnant during their teen years and menopause?

🐾 CYBILL SHEPHERD

hen it comes to pregnancy, surprises happen. We might have decided to quit having children once we turned thirty-five. Then, to our amazement, we conceived at forty. It wasn't planned. We never thought it would happen. But we are excited about the new addition, and we welcome him without hesitation. As Mary Wollstonecraft once said: "I began to love this little creature, and to anticipate his birth as a fresh twist in a knot, which I did not wish to untie."

I've had surprise parties, unannounced visits from friends, and now I get to see what little wonder the gods have bestowed on me.

241

My life, my real life, was in danger, and not from anything other people might do but from the hatred I carried in my own heart.

♪JAMES BALDWIN

A neglectful or abusive upbringing is always difficult to heal within our hearts. For years, we harbor feelings of resentment, rage, and bitterness. If we have the courage to go beneath those harsh feelings, we usually find sorrow and grief for the loss of the love we never had. As hard as it is, when we do go there, we have taken the first step in the healing process.

Having a child of our own gives us the opportunity and incentive to come to terms with our painful past. Now is the time to break free from any hatred we are carrying and to create a loving family of our own.

I will heal the demons of my past in order to become a better mother for my own child.

The real passion, not for someone. But the brief season when the exultant fact of existence courses madly through you.

✿ PATRICIA HAMPL

*I*n pregnancy, the pulse of existence courses through us. We feel part of the life cycle, and month by month we come closer to taking our place in it. No longer is life lived solely for our own purposes. We must consider the ways in which an infant will alter our household, our relationships, and the time we can dedicate to our individual dreams and pursuits. Although we might not answer all the questions or have a clear picture of what the future will bring, our passion will carry us into the next phase of motherhood.

My heart will sound out the joy of existence and the child within me will hear.

*Yes'm, old friends is always best, 'less you can catch
a new one that's fit to make an old one out of.*
🐾 SARAH ORNE JEWETT

ld friends *are* the best. They don't mind if
the house is a mess. They don't expect
pleasantries and polite service. We can be tired if
we're tired. We can act grumpy if we feel grumpy. It
doesn't matter if we're still in our robe and slippers,
having a bad hair day. They've seen our morning
face and smelled our morning breath before.

When the baby arrives, these are the friends who
will be the first to come and cook meals for the
family, wash the dishes mounting in the sink, and
rock our little one to sleep so we can curl up in bed
and get some much-needed shut-eye.

**I welcome unplanned "intrusions" from my
close, comfortable friends. They will be there
with the right assistance when I need it.**

Abundance

If you are filled with gratitude for what you have, you will feel abundant. And you cannot feel abundance and scarcity at the same time.

♫ SHARON WEGSCHEIDER-CRUSE

It's easy to get caught up in wanting our baby to have everything. We want him to have the finest clothes, the best baby furniture, organic foods, high-quality educational toys, and a trust fund to pay for an Ivy League education. When we remember the limits of our financial resources, it may be tempting to worry that our child will not have all the accoutrements of the lifestyle we would wish for him. However, if we focus on what we have instead of what we lack, we will be grateful for the abundance in our life. More important, by our example we will teach our children to do the same, thus giving them an all-important gift—the ability to be happy with what they have.

I will remember this: whatever I have to offer my child, it is enough. He will not be left wanting.

Everything and everyone is related to everything and everyone else.

🌸 MARIA HARRIS

*B*eing on the verge of motherhood changes our thoughts and behaviors. Like other mothers before us, we now turn our attention to regular feedings, breast milk, quality daycare, reliable diaper service, good school districts, and safety latches for cabinets. We have joined the inclusive club of mothers, and regardless of personality differences, parenting styles, or political affiliation, we are interconnected by virtue of our children. We know we are not the first (or the last) to contend with tender breasts and the drops of milk that form at the nipple, to make room for our ever-expanding tummy, to plan to restructure our home so it will accommodate the needs of our baby. Every day we come closer to joining the circle of mothers. We feel connected to other women, not by blood or marriage but by the weight of experience we know in our flesh.

When I feel connected to the other mothers of the world, I feel a heightened sense of belonging.

I can do anything. I have children!

🐾 BUMPER STICKER SLOGAN

*P*regnancy is a great time to grow up. It can bring out a strength we never knew we had. The heart of a lioness is forming inside of us, replacing our fear with courage. Slowly, we come to feel her power. No longer do we feel intimidated by doctors. We gather the information we need and feel confident in our ability to make our own decisions where our child is concerned. If our parents attempt to bully us into doing things their way, we tactfully let them know they have overstepped their bounds. Day by day, we feel more secure in our new role as "mother," and learn to assert ourselves in ways we never thought possible. And it's a good thing, too, for we will need all the strength we can muster for this new role.

As I prepare myself for a new role in life, I trust I will find the strength and confidence to meet whatever challenges arise.

One ought, every day at least, to hear a little song,
read a good poem, see a fine picture, and, if it were
possible, to speak a few reasonable words.
♫JOHANN WOLFGANG VON GOETHE

he poet's advice is modest, but sound. We all
need to extract ourselves from the practical
demands of each day and turn our attention toward
the inspiration around us. Whether we choose to
play classical music in the car on the way to work,
visit a museum on our lunch hour, or take a few
minutes to read words of wisdom and truth—the
point is to get a daily infusion of beauty and the
finer things in life. They will uplift us and inspire
our very souls—and help us come up with the best
we have to give.

**The practical aspects of an expectant mother's
life can consume all my attention. Now, more
than ever, it is paramount that I surround myself
with things of beauty and inspiration.**

*. . . none of my close friends had children. I felt like a
pioneer . . . the pressure was on. My comfortable
status as the family bad girl was being compromised.*
❦ ELISSA SCHAPPELL

aking the transition from party girl to new
mother is not always easy. We may have
grown accustomed to going out on Friday nights
with co-workers: soon, we will have to go straight
to the daycare center and then home to care for our
child. Instead of socializing at dinner engagements
and gallery openings, we'll be reaching for the
phone in an attempt to connect with the outside
world. It is normal to feel isolated at first and as
though we are completely "out of the loop." Yet
as our baby gets older, we may find that nights at
home intermingled with nights on the town are a
wonderful and rewarding combination.

**Becoming a mother doesn't mean I have to sud-
denly become straitlaced and boring. With the
help of grandparents and a reliable baby-sitter,
I can still go out and kick up my heels.**

Parents are the bones on which children sharpen their teeth.

🐾 PETER USTINOV

*O*nce we're on our third or fourth child, we know what to expect. We've grown accustomed to the terrible twos. When the cries of colic pierce our eardrums, we no longer panic. We know what to do. When our five-year-old totters on the balance beam at the playground, it is the young mothers who jump up as we patiently look on. We've already been broken in, so we take the mishaps in stride.

By the time my fourth child arrives, motherhood will feel as comfortable as an old pair of shoes.

Venting

I'm a venter. I have strong feelings and I vent them.

♫ LINDA D.

Some of us feel things intensely and need to vocalize our feelings. We never mean our outbursts as a personal attack. And we never mean to direct them at any one person in our family. But try as we might to control ourselves, occasionally the volume of our voice can hit decibel levels that are frightening to those around us.

It's especially important during pregnancy to find a way to manage overwhelming emotions. If we already have young children, they need a calm and comforting mom, now more than ever. Perhaps we can call a time-out for Mommy, and go to another room and call a friend who can listen until we calm down. Or we can scream into a pillow. That way, our children won't be so overwhelmed by our volatile emotions and we can protect the physical and emotional health of the little one in our belly.

When tensions build up, I need to release them. I will find constructive ways to vent my feelings without subjecting my children to them.

Bonding with Baby

From the instant I saw her, a tiny red creature bathed in the weird underwater light of the hospital operating room, I loved her with an intensity life had not prepared me for.

❧ SUSAN CHEEVER

While attachment and bonding begin during pregnancy, meeting our baby upon her birth is truly a transformative experience. Almost instantly our infant's own unique personality begins to emerge, even though we may recognize it only in retrospect. And our own personality begins to change as we make room for another loved one in our heart. The growing attachment we feel is like nothing we've ever felt before, and we know this relationship will continue to transform us for the rest of our lives.

The love I feel on meeting my baby for the first time will be truly transforming. My love for her, and hers for me, will shape both of our lives from here on.

Being an Advocate

Now that I have these children, I'm just crazed about the world's making it into the next century.

MERYL STREEP

Many of us have discovered, perhaps to our surprise, that becoming a mother means being an advocate for our children. We may have to confront teachers who will not take our child's special needs into account, or seek help for a physical or emotional problem that is out of the mainstream. We may need to put distance between ourselves and our old friends for the sake of our children. We may find we have a new appreciation for the importance of environmental, political, or other global issues. Controversies that others are ready to ignore, we must fight for. Even while our baby is still in the womb, we may need to play advocate as medical decisions are weighed. Through it all, we must find the strength to be mothers who don't take no for an answer when we know the answer should be yes!

I am prepared to fight for my children's needs. I will be their voice and their protection. No one can do that for them as well as I can.

Motherhood is the world's most intensive course in love.

♫ KATHLEEN HIRSCH AND KATRINA KENISON

Becoming a mother is one of the greatest forms of education we can receive. Every day there are profound lessons. Every day we are given tests. If we fail to learn certain lessons the first time around, we needn't worry; the topic will come up again as sure as the sun will rise and we will have another opportunity to get it right. And while parenting is the hardest course of all, it's not impossible: when our work is not satisfactory, we can redo the assignment. Fortunately, there's a great deal of room for error—if we love our children and treat them with respect, no matter how many mistakes we make, it will, in all likelihood, come out all right in the end. And if we're lucky, we'll graduate with honors.

Motherhood is an age-old doctoral program that adds challenging requirements every year. I will take my assignments seriously and do my best to keep up with the homework!

Heightened Senses

When I was pregnant, colors seemed brighter, and I felt a connectedness with other people.

         🌸 GINNY BETTENDORF

*H*eightened senses are a wonderful "side effect" of pregnancy. Flowers smell sweeter, lemons and oranges are more zesty and pungent, and the ocean spray seems to rush up like an overzealous lover stealing a salty kiss. Colors wax brighter: the pinks and gold of the sunset shimmer in the evening sky; a field of flowers makes us feel as if we've been transported to Monet's garden; and the costumes at the circus seem more vibrant and intense than ever. We have been gifted with a keen awareness of beauty and we don't want to lose it. Hopefully, we can capture it for all time.

Thanks to the child in my belly, the world around me is much more intense and beautiful. I will strive to hold on to this heightened appreciation, and pass on a joy for living to my child.

Well, if I called the wrong number, why did you answer the phone?

🐾 JAMES THURBER

*E*xpectant mothers go through phases where the things we say make no sense, and we feel like we're living in a fog. "Where did you put my car keys" we ask testily, only to discover we're holding them in our hand. "What's for dinner?" we demand, only minutes after announcing that we would be happy to prepare the evening meal. The clerk has to repeat the price of our groceries three times before we manage to coax our hand into writing a check for the correct amount. Our family is so confused by our lack of coherence they ask us to put everything in writing just in case they need to prove to us what we've said.

My mind may not be functioning at its best right now. I hope the people around me can take my incoherence in stride and laugh with me at the absurdity of my remarks.

Fatigue

Those who do not complain are never pitied.

♫ JANE AUSTEN

*F*atigue and pregnancy are a bad combination: we tend to complain about every little thing and easily find fault with those around us. We feel bad that we're so grumpy, but we can't help it. We are in serious need of a nap, but are too restless or uncomfortable to sleep. In this state, requests feel like impositions; comments are taken too personally, and we're generally out of sorts. Fortunately, our family understands. They know our bark is worse than our bite.

When I find myself turning into a curmudgeon, it's time to get out of the game and go sit on the bench.

Beware the fury of a patient man.

🌸 JOHN DRYDEN

*W*hile it is often better to hold our tongue, we'd better not hold it forever. If we have disagreements with friends, family members, or our boss, we would do well to bring the problem out into the open. Otherwise, when we least expect it, probably on a day when we're extremely tired, we will explode and blurt out more than we had intended. Why not gather up our courage and express our feelings *before* our temper flares? Otherwise, stress and tension will lodge itself in our bodies and one day, unexpectedly, explode.

Patience maintained through clenched teeth is not genuine patience. I will address the issues that aggravate me before they get out of hand.

Changing One's Mind

I didn't want to know the sex of my child until I came across these adorable matching mother-daughter purses.

👣 BETSY ALLEN

The funniest things can make us change our mind when it comes to knowing the sex of our child in advance. My friend Betsy, like many new mothers, wanted it to be a surprise. For the longest time maintaining the mystery was more important than knowing what colors to decorate the nursery, which clothes to buy, or whether she needed to be picking a girl's or a boy's name.

Then, without warning, a silly little item in a local shop made her change her mind completely. As it turned out, her baby was a girl—so she was able to justify buying the matching purses before her daughter exited the womb.

Pregnancy is an unpredictable time. I will allow myself to change my mind, and will enjoy the changes.

Be not angry that you cannot make others as you wish them to be, since you cannot make yourself as you wish to be.

🎵 THOMAS À KEMPIS

t is all too easy to project our own unfulfilled wishes onto our unborn child. "I hope she doesn't have my short temper," we think. Or "I hope he is taller than my husband and won't go bald in his thirties." In short, we hope that our child will possess all the traits we see as "good" and none of the ones we deem "bad." But just as we have imperfections and disagreeable traits, so will our children. We would do well to remember that we can love both ourselves and our children without liking every single characteristic.

If I expect myself to be perfect, I will expect my child to be perfect. That's a surefire recipe for disappointment. Acceptance of ourselves and of our children for who they are is the key to happiness.

. . . with calm mind embrace, thou fool, a rest that knows no care.

🌺 LUCRETIUS

*W*hy is it that we feel guilty when we nap? Are we afraid that the chores left undone will multiply and we'll be set back even further if we don't keep in constant motion? Even when we're pregnant, we feel we need a doctor's orders to justify resting our head on a pillow and closing our eyes. We're so accustomed to being indispensable that we fear the world might collapse if we drift off for thirty minutes. When we're carrying a baby, one of our most important duties is to stay healthy and rested. So when the voice of guilt kicks in, there is only one appropriate response: "Shhh! Mommy's resting. . . ."

My baby needs me to stay rested and strong. I will be sure to schedule time to be carried away to dreamland.

A friend of mine calls the most difficult part of birth "Labor Land": the stretch of time when your entire reality is composed of contractions—the one you just had, the one you're having now, and the one you're anticipating. It usually strikes just before the pushing stage when you're almost—almost—completely dilated.

🐾 ANN-MARIE GIGLIO

*I*f our mate learns only one thing in childbirth class, it should be this: "Labor Land" is when we need him the most. During transition, we can become overwhelmed by the intensity of the experience and may feel like we're "losing it." We may scream or moan or hurl verbal attacks. If our partner becomes impatient with us, shows the sheer terror on his face (making us feel even more uncertain), or passes out, he will compound the problem. If, on the other hand, he is calm, connected, and lovingly supportive during this difficult stage of labor, he will give us the faith and endurance we need to reach the next phase, when the midwife finally says, "Push!"

I will help prepare my labor coach for what is to come, and will ask him or her to stay with me and remain calm, even when I am out of control.

The more people have studied different methods of bringing up children, the more they have come to the conclusion that what good mothers and fathers instinctively feel like doing for their babies is the best after all.

♫ BENJAMIN SPOCK

*E*xpectant mothers have a lot of new information thrown in their direction. Some of that information comes from authorities who have years of experience behind them. While it is important to listen to what others tell us about the risks involved in childbirth, health concerns, diet, and infant care, we would do well to withhold our final decisions. After we've gathered up sufficient information, we can take time to reflect on the choices that are most fitting for us and our baby. This is good practice for being a parent—an endeavor that often involves making decisions in situations where what's right and what's wrong is not at all clear.

As a parent I have to learn to make the best decisions I can without always knowing whether I've done "the right thing."

*Who knows what women can be when they are
finally free to become themselves?*

🌸 BETTY FRIEDAN

*J*t is an exciting time to be a woman. Even the
role of motherhood is experiencing a rebirth;
we no longer have only two choices—stay-at-home
mom or working professional mother—but a whole
range of options that were inconceivable just a few
decades ago. We can work from home and telecom-
mute while our children are playing at a neighborhood daycare center or in the next room with a
baby-sitter. Or we could start our own business—
selling toys and children's apparel or providing
child care to others—so there is little separation
between our job and our mothering responsibilities.
We can work as freelancers, or take advantage of
the growing opportunities for part-time and flex-
time arrangements. Or we can trade childcare shifts
with our spouses. In other words, our choices are
as endless as our own capacity to imagine.

**Being myself is one of the greatest contributions
I can make to my family. My whole family will
benefit if I create a lifestyle in which my top
priorities are in harmony with my everyday life.**

How glorious it is, but how painful it is also, to be exceptional in this world!

👣 ALFRED DE MUSSET

Some of us felt misunderstood by our parents. They never seemed to "get" what we were saying. They didn't make the same intellectual leaps we did, or furrow their brows over the pressing questions of existence like we did. They loved us, yet they did not attempt to meet us in our world.

As we prepare for motherhood, it's fun to fantasize about the activities we will want to share with our child. But it will be even more important to remain open to the interests she will introduce us to. Not only will this lead us into wonderful new life experiences we can't even imagine, it will assure her that we love her for the unique being she is. That's a great gift for any child!

I will celebrate my child's unique qualities as soon as I discover what they are. Together we will explore the world through her eyes.

The first and great commandment is, Don't let them scare you.

♫ ELMER DAVIS

*I*f we haven't already heard all the birthing horror stories, we surely will. Why is it that mothers latch onto us and share the gory details of their labor? Perhaps they see it as their duty to let us know what delivering a baby is *really* like. Whatever the reason, they usually do more harm than good. First of all, since every birth is a completely unique experience, the stories of other births have very little to do with what we are about to experience. Second, there is more than likely a correlation between bad experiences and eager storytellers. The contented moms are happy to keep their stories close to their hearts—and to allow us to have our own experience.

Birthing horror stories can conjure up needless fears and worries. I will avoid those women who insist on telling their tales to reluctant listeners.

"You are the caretaker of the generations, you are the birth giver," the Sun told the woman. "You will be the carrier of this universe."

❀ SUN CREATION MYTH OF THE BRULÉ SIOUX

*A*t times, we feel the huge responsibility of becoming a mother. It is indeed a sacred responsibility, a profound initiation that cannot be undertaken lightly. In order to perform the tasks of motherhood, we must prepare not only our homes but our hearts and minds as well. It's true: the next generation depends on us. That's a big role to fill—and one that is impossible to be really ready for. But we can grow into it, one day at a time.

I will reflect on the awesome responsibilities of becoming a mother and will embrace them with honor as they are bestowed on me.

The state of being pregnant [is] as if you're weaving
a house for your child out of your own body, and it
takes all your energy, all your attention.

🐾 HILMA WOLITZER

e can be moving through our day when
suddenly it hits us: we're doing something
miraculous. A baby is growing inside of us and with
our own blood and nutrients; we are providing him
with everything he needs to become a complete
human being. With that in mind, it is obviously
important to keep fit. Studies show that women
who exercise regularly and take time to stretch and
loosen their muscles tend to have an easier pregnancy and birth. The benefits far outweigh the has-
sle of putting on a bathing suit or running pants. If
we don't feel motivated to exercise on our own we
can join a pregnancy exercise class at the local
recreation center and enjoy the socializing as well
as the exercise. After all, we are "weaving a house"
for our little one. For both our sakes, the house
should be strong and solid!

There is no substitute for safe exercise during
pregnancy. I will take good care of myself during
this special time.

No matter how many licenses we issue or inspections we require, no matter how rigid the guidelines we establish or how much money we pay, we must face the fact that it is impossible to have quality controls over the capacity of one human being to love and care for another.

♪ LINDA BURTON

First impressions are not always accurate. Make sure, when choosing a nanny or baby nurse, that the person has a personality compatible with yours. Take time to discuss your thoughts about the care of a newborn to see if you share the same views. Watch how she interacts with your older children, your pets, and other members of your family. Pay attention to your instinctive reactions —do you find an instant sense of trust and confidence in her or are you plagued by vague but insistent doubts? After all, hiring someone who will be sharing the responsibility not only for your newborn but for your entire family is an intimate collaboration. You want to make sure she is a good fit.

I will take time to get to know my nanny before hiring her on a permanent basis. That way, we can see if we are truly compatible.

Impulses

The Devil made me buy that dress!

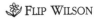 FLIP WILSON

*I*n the last month of pregnancy, most of us can't wait to fit back into our old clothes. We fantasize about having our body back, walking down the street in a slinky dress and high heels. We have a waist, normal-sized breasts, and a tight behind. And if we happen to pass a gorgeous dress in a department store window today, we might just buy it—in our usual size, of course!

My new dress will help motivate me, turning fantasies into reality after the birth of my baby.

Tubs of flowers were always moved inside the birth room on the principle . . . that the first things the eye of a newborn saw should be beautiful.

🐾 NORMAN RUSH

*W*hether we give birth in a hospital or in our own home, it's nice to create an atmosphere of beauty and tranquility if we can. We can arrange flowers in a vase, light candles, or burn essential oils to soothe the senses. We can play beautiful music. That way, our infant's first experience of the world will be special and sacred, and his departure from the safety of the womb will not be so abrupt.

If possible, I will decorate the birthing room so my infant's first view of the world will be a warm and welcoming one.

Clumsiness

America is a large, friendly dog in a very small room.
Every time it wags its tail it knocks over a chair.

♫ ARNOLD TOYNBEE

*I*sn't this a wonderful description? Doesn't it seem to fit us during the final months of pregnancy? No matter how high we carry our baby, our stomachs are always getting in the way. At work, we bend over the Xerox machine to make copies and other employees can't pass by without pressing their backs against the wall. On the subway, we say, "Excuse me," repeatedly, as we bump into fellow commuters. Although we always try to be pleasant about it, the fact remains: our tummies bump into things and occasionally knock things over.

Doubling my width can increase the chances of clumsiness. But I can be friendly about it.

Two new people were born in that moment. Justin was born . . . and I was reborn. . . . Gone was the self-centered twenty-three-year-old student, more still a girl than a woman. I had labored to bring a child into the world, and the fear and pain I suffered had somehow awakened a new compassion in my heart

❦ JOAN BORYSENKO

*B*irthing a baby changes us forever. In a few hours' time we cross the threshold into the mysteries and profound responsibilities of womanhood, and there is no turning back. And while some of us adapt more quickly to the change than others, we all respond to the call. It doesn't matter if the changes show on the outside, we feel them on the inside. No longer are our thoughts consumed by our own cares. We must now think for two and be mature enough to make adult decisions.

I will embrace the profound changes that motherhood brings and welcome the initiation into the mysteries of womanhood.

There aren't any words yet invented to define the emotions a mother feels as she cuddles her newborn child.

JANET LEIGH

oy, happiness, ecstasy, fulfillment, love, abundance, bliss . . . Try as we might to put our feelings into words to those friends who have not become mothers, we always come up short. Being pregnant and giving birth are experiences a person must go through in order to fully understand them. They are so unlike anything else that others really cannot comprehend the journey unless they, too, experience it.

The experience of becoming a new mother is indescribable. I will speak from my heart even though my words may be inadequate to capture the intensity of it.

Opening and closing the front door soundlessly, an art known to mothers of sleeping babies. . . .

♫ ELIZABETH CUNNINGHAM

*I*f we haven't already mastered the art of closing doors soundlessly, we'd better start practicing. The careless slam of a door while our newborn is napping could spoil our plans to make a phone call, browse through a magazine, finish a nap, or scrub the toilet. As new mothers learn, babies have keen radar. They sense our every move. They know when we are coming and going. They know when we are trying to get something accomplished—and they hate to miss out on anything!

I must learn new ways of doing things. I will practice being quiet as a mouse, or maybe just enjoy not having to do so—yet!

Surprises and Adjustments

Everyone told me that I was carrying a boy. They insisted that the little protrusion on the ultrasound was a penis. Who was I to argue? They were the experts. Some experts! My "little boy" was actually a girl that had a habit of sticking her fingers between her legs.

        ⚓ NANCY GOLDMAN

*O*ne of the biggest surprises of pregnancy can be finding out on the delivery table that after all this time, when you thought you were having a boy, a baby girl had popped out! Even when we "know" the gender of our child in advance, it might be better to save purchasing gender-specific baby clothes until after the birth. Because mistakes are made. And though we've come a long way toward neutralizing sex-role stereotypes, most parents aren't comfortable dressing their little girls in football jerseys or their little boys in pink. As for the shock—well, as new parents we already have a million adjustments to make, so what's one more?

I will prepare myself for a life full of surprises and adjustments—some of them rather large— and will do my best to take it all in stride.

What do we live for, if it is not to make life less difficult for each other?

GEORGE ELIOT

sn't it wonderful when our little ones rest their heads on our tummies to listen to the sounds of their little brother or sister? Including our older children in our pregnancies allows them to feel part of something very important, instead of feeling as though they are left out of the big event. They can feel secure in our love even though, in a short while, they will have to share it.

I will make sure all my children know they can bask in the warmth of my love. Like the eternal sunshine, there's always enough love to go around.

I can still remember rocking them to sleep on my lap in the middle of the night, to soothe them back to sleep after a stomach ache or a bad dream, the songs I would make up. . . .

♪ BETTY FRIEDAN

*L*ullabies are a balm for the heart. The sweet melody soothes our baby while we rock her gently to sleep. A favorite lullaby can comfort our child when she is in need. Even the silly songs we make up can carry her to dreamland.

Babies are able to hear by the fifth month of pregnancy. If we start to sing to them in utero, the melodies we sing to them later will provide them with a vital and deeply comforting connection to their days in the womb.

I will sing sweet lullabies to my child so that when she arrives, she will remember the tunes from her peaceful days in the womb.

Using the oar as a kind of listening straw, you can hear the sounds of the underwater world. Some fish are a noisy lot. Sea robins, drum-fishes and many others make sounds with their swim bladders; croakers grunt loud enough to keep China Sea fishermen awake at night; Hawaiian triggerfish grind their teeth loudly; the male toad-fish growls; bottlenose dolphins click and squeak like badly oiled office chairs; bowhead whales purr and twirp; humpback whales put on a songfest.

🐚 DIANE ACKERMAN

*W*e tend to think of being underwater as a silent experience. Yet water amplifies sound and bends it into new shapes for our listening ear.

Just think of all the fascinating sounds our growing baby is hearing in her watery bower: digestive gurgles, the thumps and echoes of our beating heart, murmurs of songs, sniffles and laughs and sneezes. Our womb must be a symphony of sound! However, honking horns and loud, angry voices also resonate in our body. For both of your sakes, why not take some time every day to listen to Jewel, Mozart, or Ella Fitzgerald, perhaps?

Both my baby and I benefit whenever we are surrounded by soothing sounds.

Babies are born wizened with instinct. They know in their bones what is right and what to do about it.

🐾 CLARISSA PINKOLA ESTES

*B*abies know what they want and they come into the world prepared to get it. When they are hungry, they cry. When they are uncomfortable, they squirm. When they want to be cuddled, they wail. They do not apologize for their needs. They do not ask others' permission to have them. They know, in their bones, to ask for what they want.

How long has it been since we felt free enough to ask that our needs be met? Or do we make up excuses for ignoring them, thinking we can "tough it out?" Perhaps we can learn from our little ones to ask for what we need.

The demands of motherhood are overwhelming. I need to take some time to reconnect with myself so I can ask for the help, the reassurance, and whatever else I need.

[Motherhood] humbled my ego and stretched my soul. It awakened me to eternity. It made me know my own humanity, my own mortality, my own limits. It gave me whatever crumbs of wisdom I possess today.

♫ ERICA JONG

*D*o we feel ready for motherhood? Have we taken the time to consider how profound the changes will be? Have we invited friends to share in the epiphanies we are having? Have we taken time to talk to our mothers and grandmothers, to ask them to share their wisdom and experience with us? If not, now is the time. Those who have already become mothers have much wisdom to impart if we will only listen.

I will join the circle of mothers by benefiting from their wisdom, by hearing their stories and listening to the passages they've experienced. It will make me a better mother.

. . . a baby . . . puts its arms around your neck and presses its hot cheek against you as it falls asleep, convinced all will be well when it wakes.

❦ ALICE HOFFMAN

The idea of having another human being who is so dependent on us can be unnerving. Sometimes we are at ease with the knowledge that we are the adults and the responsibility falls to us. At other times, we may feel panicked at the very thought. To our child, it doesn't matter how much we doubt ourselves as we come to terms with the responsibility of motherhood. When he puts his arms around our neck and presses his hot cheek against us, he has no doubt that we can rise to the occasion.

My child may have more confidence in me than I sometimes do. I will grow to be worthy of his trust.

When Mommy was pregnant with you and looked like a cow, I told her she was beautiful 'cos I didn't want to hurt her feelings.

JIM CARREY, IN *LIAR, LIAR*

Pregnant women are not fat. And in no way do we resemble our bovine friends in the fields. We are round and luscious, voluptuous and full. If others insist on watching our weight for us, concerned that we may not return to being our "glamorous, svelte" selves, we should ignore their worries and do what we know is right for the baby. After all, we don't need two people hawking the scales!

I must not allow others to make me self-conscious or ashamed during pregnancy. I will take pride in the fullness of my body.

I think it pisses God off if you walk by the color purple in a field somewhere and don't notice it.

♫ ALICE WALKER

$\mathcal{P}$regnancy opens our eyes to beauty in a new way. Our spirit comes alive and the colors of the world flood into view. Things we had walked right past only a few days earlier now tap us on the shoulder, demanding that we delight in their majesty. Flowers beckon us to gaze on them. We notice beautifully woven baskets in craft-shop windows; we see that the leaves in the trees are vibrant green; we appreciate the sensual formation of rocks that look sculpted by God himself.

We must not forget to look at ourselves with the same loving eyes. Are we not a creation of God, full of God's wonderful creation?

The miracle of new life is one of God's finest creations. We must open our eyes to that miracle within us.

*Lamaze is great and the classes totally educated
Pammy and me about what to expect, but I never
intended to have a natural childbirth. The moment
epidurals were mentioned in our class, Pammy and I
turned to each other and nodded.*

❦ ANNE LAMOTT

hile it is important to weigh the pros and
cons of various birthing methods, it is best
not to allow others to make this decision for us. Just
because we had a C-section with our first child
doesn't automatically mean we have to have
another with our second. Plenty of women have
V-BACs: vaginal birth after cesarean. If induced
labor is recommended and we are uncomfortable
with that advice, we might request that another
doctor in our healthcare program examine us. If our
closest friend had a natural birth, but we have a low
threshold of pain and don't think that's for us, we
will want to explore other options with our obstetrician ahead of time.

**I will be honest with myself about choosing
which birthing method is most comfortable
for me.**

Living well is the best revenge.

👣 GEORGE HERBERT

*M*any of us are on our second marriage. Perhaps our former partner didn't want children; perhaps he would have been an uninvolved father. Maybe he treated us badly and we decided against having children with him. If we left an abusive situation to start fresh, it is likely that we felt bitter and angry at first; betrayed, because things had not turned out the way we had hoped. Now is a good time to let go of any leftover feelings of anger and bitterness.

After all, we did find someone we *can* share our life with; someone who wants to have children. There should be no more need for thoughts of revenge—they will be crowded out by gratitude for the wonderful new life we have now.

The only revenge that is truly sweet is leaving bitterness behind to find true love. I am thankful for the new partner I have found to share the joy of raising a family together.

Stop the World—I Want to Get Off
♫ ANTHONY NEWLY AND LESLIE BRICUSSE

*W*e've all had days when it feels like the world is spinning too fast for us to keep up. All we want to do is get off for a while. The next time we feel this way, we might want to consider calling in sick for a day or scheduling a three-day weekend so we can look forward to a mini-vacation. If we have some unused vacation time, why not get an e-ticket to Mexico, Hawaii, or the Caribbean? After all, it may be our last time to travel without a baby in tow for several years to come.

I may not be able to leave the planet, but I can certainly escape to a lovelier spot.

*A rock pile ceases to be a rock pile the moment a
single man contemplates it, bearing within him the
image of a cathedral.*

🐚 ANTOINE DE SAINT-EXUPÉRY

*I*t is easy to become focused on the different
scenarios of what birth will be like for *us*. Yet
if we take a moment to think about our baby and
the ordeal she will go through just to gasp her first
breath, we realize how intense birth is for *her*. She
will be violently pushed out of her home and
squeezed down a dark canal. At times she may feel
trapped and her heart may race. Luckily, we will be
waiting for her with open arms on the other end
and will be there to reassure her that all will be well
in this strange new world.

**I will remember to be present for myself *and* my
baby during the birth process. If I keep her and
her needs clearly in mind, I will be better able to
get through my own experience.**

The worst part of success is to try finding someone who is happy for you.

🦶 BETTE MIDLER

hy is it that some people try to cut us down when we are at our most successful and most vibrant? If we find ourselves around old friends who are threatened by our success or happiness, or who are unable to be supportive, it is time to find a new set of friends, friends who will encourage us in our new avenues of growth. There's no need for confrontation—we can quietly put our energies in a new direction and hope our old friends will catch up with us again someday.

I will not sacrifice my newfound happiness because others cannot enjoy it with me. I will choose friends who support the paths I choose.

*Birth is like a marriage. You have to know what you
want but be prepared for anything.*

♫ ANONYMOUS

*I*n birth, the unexpected is normal. Rarely do
deliveries go exactly as planned. Little
glitches arise and we must respond to each one
as needed. A fetal distress signal may alter plans
for a home birth. Contractions that are steadily
coming closer and closer together can slow down
or stop and oxytocin may be needed to get labor
moving again.

Certainly, it helps to know what kind of birth
we want, but at the same time, it helps to stay
flexible and expect the unexpected.

**Giving birth is one of the most unpredictable
experiences in life. I will remain open to
alterations during its course.**

The statistics on sanity are that one out of every four Americans is suffering from some form of mental illness. Think of your three best friends. If they're okay, then it's you.

🌸 RITA MAE BROWN

*D*uring pregnancy, fluctuating hormones can make us feel as though we're losing our marbles. We become irrationally upset over the strangest things: a traffic light that takes too long to change, a difficult meeting at work, a dirty pan left in the sink. We don't seem to have the ability to cope with the normal ups and downs of life as well as we used to, and we're often on the verge of tears without even knowing why. Are we losing our minds or regressing to an infantile state? No, we are simply expectant mothers riding the roller coaster of our emotions.

When it feels as though I'm losing my grip, I'll remind myself to hang on tight—this is all part of the roller-coaster ride known as pregnancy.

Is it really so difficult to tell a good action from a bad one? I think one usually knows right away or a moment afterward, in a horrid flash of regret.
🐾 MARY MCCARTHY

*E*ver notice how, when we close our eyes in a certain way, it enables us to take a deep breath and regroup in stressful situations? It's our body's way of helping us to reflect, even if it takes less than a minute. Our body gives us a moment to regain our composure so we can act with more clarity and patience. For example, if a coworker puts us down, instead of reacting, we can close our eyes and wait a few seconds before we respond. This will give us a chance to choose our words more carefully and avoid saying something we'll regret.

Closing our eyes to look better into ourselves is a wonderful technique to put into practice during pregnancy.

I will close my eyes and take a deep breath whenever I feel like I'm at the end of my rope and about to react.

*It was easy in those uncomplicated days, to treat our
as-yet-unborn children as the parentheses in the
otherwise fascinating narrative of our life stories.*

♫ LINDA BURTON

*B*efore we conceived, life with a child always
seemed uncomplicated when we thought
about it in the abstract. But now, as we approach
the final weeks of pregnancy, we are beginning to
get a realistic glimpse of what it actually takes to be
a parent. Instead of folding neatly into our life, our
child will more than likely disrupt and alter it.
Rather than going along with the plans we have
charted out, he will come equipped with his own
agenda. Luckily, as adults, we can construct the
framework. However, it must be pliable enough to
bend with the needs of our child.

**I cannot foresee the specific changes my child
will bring, but I will be open to embracing her as
part of my new life.**

Nothing happens, nobody comes, nobody goes, it's awful!

🌸 SAMUEL BECKETT

*D*uring the days surrounding our due date, we often feel like we're "waiting for Godot." The monotony of pregnancy sets in and we feel like we're in terminal stasis. One hour runs into the next. We're bored. We want to get on with it. But the days crawl by, eon by eon, until the tension is almost unbearable. Then, finally, our contractions begin and the waiting is suddenly over. We're on our way. . . .

People always tell me how hard the birthing process is, but the waiting can be harder.

Sleep faster, we need the pillows.

🦶 JEWISH PROVERB

*T*he final month of pregnancy can be a real challenge for husbands. Even if they snore, rarely can they drown out the complaints of a pregnant woman who groans like a horse with colic. As hard as we try, we can't find a comfortable position in bed. We toss and turn. We stuff a pillow between our legs, hoping to ease the discomfort of our knees pressing together, only to end up asking our husband for his. If we're lucky enough to find a halfway decent position and finally settle in, our bladder cries out: "Get me to the toilet!" If our husbands are serious about getting any sleep themselves, they'd better flop on the couch.

I'll most likely be adjusting and readjusting my position in bed during the final month of pregnancy. My cat may be the only bed companion who stays with me.

Traditions are the guideposts driven deep into our subconscious minds. The most powerful ones are those we can't even describe, aren't even aware of.

♪ ELLEN GOODMAN

*W*hen considering a name for our first child, we might not have to look farther than our own family. If, for instance, all boys have been named after their father, and all girls have carried their mother's name, or a variation thereof, we know what our decision will be. In keeping with family tradition, we will pass on our family names and our child will carry the rich lineage of those who came before him.

My child will carry the family name, just as I did, and my mother before me.

I am a restlessness inside a stillness inside a restlessness.
✿ DODIE SMITH

*O*ften, right before giving birth, we experience a restless period. We can't sit still and we become compulsive nesters. We are impatient with everyone and we may snap at our mate. Luckily, our husbands turn the other cheek. They understand the stresses of pregnancy and easily forgive our transgressions. They offer foot rubs. They hold our hands and kiss our foreheads, helping to calm us down.

Restless agitation is common during the final month of pregnancy. With support and understanding, I will get through it.

. . . the word most common to children's speech, most often called out, most repeated for comfort, is "Mommy." I have never known a mother to feel besmirched by this—harassed, yes; but degraded? Nonsense.

🐾 SONIA JOHNSON

eady or not, here it comes. We will be trailed by the word "Mommy" for the rest of our lives. When our child falls out of the apple tree, it is "Mommy" she will call for first. When she is proud of a new accomplishment, she will call out "Watch me, Mommy!" When she is in need of comfort, when she can't find us, when she is perplexed by the behavior of strangers, when the noises at the mall or on the street overwhelm her, she will call out to us. "Mommy" will be her mantra and her lifeline.

How exciting to think that soon *I* will be *"The Mommy."*

I had no doubt I would go back to work after the baby was born. Throughout all nine months of pregnancy I assured everyone that I was not a "homebody," that I'd be bored at home, and that I needed to be out in the world. Then she was born. The nurse brought this small, soft, warm baby to me, and I immediately fell deeply in love.

♫ PAM SVOBODA

Sound familiar? Many of us who are first-time, working-outside-the-home mothers probably feel the same way Pam did. We're certain we'll return to work shortly after the birth of our child. But what if our feelings change? What if we decide we want to spend more time at home than originally planned? Are we prepared financially to manage such a change of heart? If not, we might want to think about putting some money away for monthly expenses so that we're better able to make a final decision that accommodates both our heart's desires and our economic realities.

Saving money for the future is a good idea. Now that I'm pregnant, it's an even better one.

*My husband is a college professor. After he teaches,
he gets to come home to our baby while I have to wait
until 6:00 P.M. I feel like I'm missing out.*
🌸 CAROLINE TWAIN

*O*ur work schedules dominate our lives. However, that doesn't mean we can't request changes in the schedule when our life changes. What about asking to work at home a couple of days a week? Or leaving early so we can be sure to get home in time to nurse our child during the dinner hour? Or bringing Baby to work with us once in a while, or even on a regular basis? There are a myriad of creative solutions to the problem of "not enough time" to be with our kids, if we make this concern a priority.

**Even before the birth, I will try to negotiate
changes in my work schedule that will allow
me time to be with my new baby.**

Great teachers empathize with kids, respect them and believe that each one has something special that can be built upon.

🐾 ANN LIEBERMAN

*R*emember your favorite teachers or college professors? Why were they your favorites? Because they believed in you. They built on your strengths. They helped you overcome your weaknesses. They listened when you talked and they showed you respect even when they corrected your behavior.

One of the most important jobs a mother has is to teach. Our child will look to us for guidance, knowledge, and wisdom. When she makes a mistake, we will be there to help her learn a better way. When she reaches a milestone, we will be there to cheer her on. Like all good teachers, we will believe in her and will always be on her side.

Thinking about my favorite teachers helps me to envision the type of mother I would like to be. I will do my best to follow in their footsteps.

I felt threatened by my husband's bottle-feeding my child. I wanted her all to myself.

♫ KATIE TAYLOR

hen we're pregnant, we picture ourselves becoming closer than ever to our mate. However, once the baby arrives, we may experience emotions we would have never expected: jealousy, possessiveness, or selfishness. We want to bond with our infant so completely that our mate's attempts to involve himself are seen as an intrusion.

While it's natural that we want our baby all to ourselves, it's important to give our husband time to bond with the baby, too. Otherwise, when we *do* want to leave the house by ourselves (and be assured, we will), our infant will pitch a fit. If Daddy is basically a stranger, we'll be so upset by our infant's cries when we try to go out that we will forfeit our alone time. And if this becomes a habit, the whole family will suffer.

I trust that my bond with my child will be secure. I will not have to force it along by being overly possessive. And I want our baby to have a good relationship with his father, too.

It takes a village to raise a child.
🌸 AFRICAN PROVERB

In many parts of the world, childbirth is a community event. New mothers are cared for by the members of an extended family, and the thought of a mother going back to work full-time when her baby is just a few weeks old is unheard of. Even in some modern, industrialized countries, mothers of young children are given as much as several *years* to devote to the all-consuming task of caring for them.

Wouldn't it be wonderful if mothers in the United States were given the same opportunity to recuperate from the birth and adjust to having a new baby in the house, with plenty of helping hands to share the burden? While we can't expect to change our society overnight, we might incorporate some of the wise practices other cultures use to ease the transition into parenthood. Perhaps close friends, or their children, need some part-time work—and could be enlisted to help with the cleaning, playing with older children, or walking the dog.

If I plan ahead, and allow friends and family to help me, I can be assured of a smooth recovery.

. . . there was something so blissful about smelling the top of a baby's head, like becoming clean and new again yourself, getting a chance to do it over. . . .

GAIL GODWIN

There is nothing like a newborn to remind us of the beauty of new beginnings. Even if the wrinkles on their little faces look remarkably like the markings of an old soul, their fresh scent reminds us that they have come straight from God. In their presence we feel as though life has begun again. We are filled with optimism. We see the wondrous possibilities of life and notice doors opening all around us.

Certain doors may close as a result of motherhood, yet new doors that I could never have imagined or hoped for will open. I will walk through them. I am ready.

Anderson, Peggy. *Great Quotes from Great Women.*
Franklin Lakes, NJ: Career Press, 1997.

Barron, James Douglas. *She's Having a Baby and
I'm Having a Breakdown.* New York: William
Morrow, 1998.

Burton, Linda, Janet Dittmer, and Cheri Loveless.
*What's a Smart Woman Like You Doing at
Home?* Washington, DC: Acropolis Books,
1986.

Carola, Leslie, ed. *Motherhood: Quotes from and
About Mothers.* Stamford, CT: Longmeadow
Press, 1992.

Exley, Helen. *A Special Collection in Praise of
Mothers.* New York: Exley Publications, 1995.

Giglio, Ann-Marie, ed. *Labor Day: Shared
Experiences from the Delivery Room.* New
York: Workman Publishing, 1999.

Handley, Helen and Andra Samuelson, eds. *Child: A
Literary Companion.* New York: Pushcart
Press, 1992.

Ingelman-Sundberg, Axel. *A Child Is Born: The
Drama of Life Before Birth.* New York: Dell
Publishing, 1965.

Klaus, Marshall H., and Phyllis H. Klaus. *Your
Amazing Newborn.* Cambridge, MA: Perseus
Books, 1998.

Kline, Christina Baker, ed. *Child of Mine: Writers Talk About the First Year of Motherhood.* New York: Dell Publishing, 1997.

Lerner, Harriet. *The Mother Dance: How Children Change Your Life.* New York: HarperCollins, 1998.

Louden, Jennifer. *The Pregnant Woman's Comfort Book.* San Francisco: HarperCollins, 1995.

McFadden, Tara Ann, ed., and Carrie Fisher. *Mothers: A Loving Celebration.* Philadelphia: Running Press, 1997.

Partnow, Elaine, ed. *The New Quotable Women.* New York: Penguin Books, 1992.

The Quotable Women. Ontario: Running Press, 1991.

Shellenbarger, Sue. *Work & Family. Essays from the "Work & Family" column of the Wall Street Journal.* New York: Ballantine, 1999.

Sorel, Nancy Caldwell, ed. *Ever Since Eve: Personal Reflections on Childbirth.* New York: Oxford University Press, 1984.

Stoddard, Alexandra. *Mothers: A Celebration.* New York: Avon Books, 1996.

Tilsner, Julie. *Planet Parenthood: Adapting to Your New Life Form.* Chicago: NTC/Contemporary Books, 2000.